THE FABULOUS
fifties

THE FABULOUS *fifties*

When Life Really Begins:
Interviews with Australian Women in Their Fifties

✣✣✣

JAN BOWEN

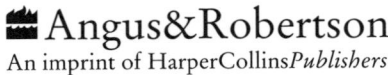
Angus&Robertson
An imprint of HarperCollins*Publishers*

ACKNOWLEDGMENTS

As well as the nine wonderful women who made this book what it is, sincere thanks is due to Margaret Coleman, yet another 'fabulous fifty' who spent so many hours plugged into the dictaphone typing the records of interview.

Angus&Robertson
An imprint of HarperCollins*Publishers*, Australia

First published in Australia in 1995

Copyright © Jan Bowen 1995

This book is copyright.
Apart from any fair dealing for the purposes of
private study, research, criticism or review,
as permitted under the Copyright Act, no part
may be reproduced by any process without written permission.
Inquiries should be addressed to the publishers.

HarperCollins*Publishers*
25 Ryde Road, Pymble, Sydney NSW 2073, Australia
31 View Road, Glenfield, Auckland 10, New Zealand
77–85 Fulham Palace Road, London W6 8JB, United Kingdom
Hazelton Lanes, 55 Avenue Road, Suite 2900, Toronto, Ontario M5R 3L2
and 1995 Markham Road, Scarborough, Ontario M1B 5M8, Canada
10 East 53rd Street, New York NY 10032, USA

National Library of Australia Cataloguing-in-Publication data:

Bowen, Jan
The fabulous fifties: when life really begins:
interviews with Australian women in their fifties.
ISBN 0 207 18653 7.
1.Middle-aged women — Australia — Interviews. 2.Middle-aged women — Australia — Biography. I.Title.
305.420994

Printed by Griffin Press

9 8 7 6 5 4 3 2 1
99 98 97 96 95

Contents

Introduction 7

Sara Henderson 13

Wendy McCarthy 27

Kendra Sundquist 43

Eve Mahlab 59

Anne Ferguson 71

Nene King 87

Helen Leonard 101

Quentin Bryce 117

Jeannette McHugh 131

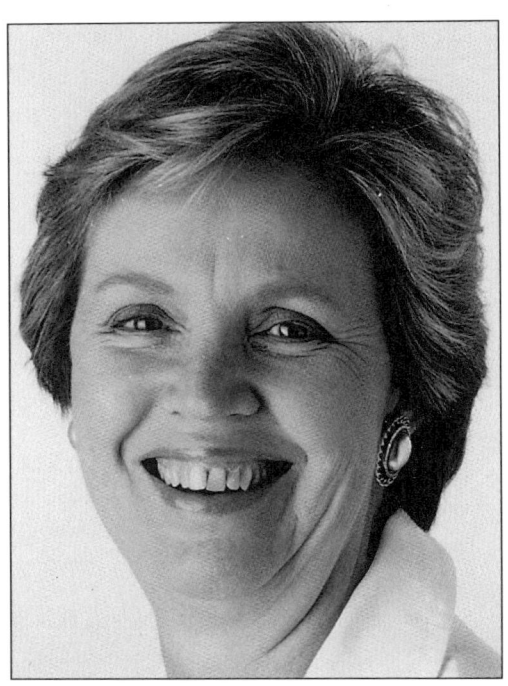

JAN BOWEN

Introduction

Twenty. Thirty. Forty. Fifty! For most people, each decade is a landmark, when we leave behind one era and pass into a new one. It is a time of analysis and reassessment, sometimes detailed and in-depth, in an effort to bring about change, sometimes merely cursory, noting only a slightly more than usually significant anniversary.

Turning fifty tends to be a particular milestone, and not always a welcome one. In this society which so glorifies youth, at fifty it cannot be denied that we are no longer young. In this society which equates beauty with youth, suddenly we are confronted with impending physical decline, an implied fading of attractiveness, of sexuality. In this society which treats youth and sexuality as a woman's main assets, women especially are valued less and less as they get older.

But at fifty, increasing life expectancy means that most of us have at least three and possibly four decades still before us. Measured in terms of total life span, we may have fewer years ahead than are already past since we are, as yet, unlikely to live until we reach one hundred. But in terms of adult life, from when we reach maturity and our life becomes 'ours', and our responsibility, we are barely half-way there. Most of us would count our mature years from thirty on, and we are only two decades past that. We may have twice that much still to come. Life expectancy for women is now eighty years of age and it has been estimated that one-third of people now in their forties will live until they are ninety. Measured according to that yardstick, we have at least as much and probably a great deal more living still to do than we have done already.

Author of the 1970s' ground-breaking best seller, *Passages*, Gail Sheehy has described the fifties as the 'youth of a woman's Second Adulthood' and there seems every reason to accept her definition. First there is childhood and the teenage years and then there is the First Adulthood from about twenty-five to forty-five. At fifty, we are entering on a new phase, a time to establish new ground rules and set the pattern for the next thirty or forty years.

What are the things that distinguish the fifties from earlier decades?

For women, the fifties are marked by obvious physical change. Menopause means the end of their reproductive life, sometimes accompanied by uncomfortable, even distressing physical symptoms, but also, more often than not, heralding a new freedom when hormonal fluctuations have ceased to impact on day-to-day living.

At fifty, many people are moving towards the conclusion of their working life. Some are looking forward to it with eager anticipation and will grasp the nettle early, leaving the workforce a mere five years later, taking the early retirement so often made available at fifty-five, to develop or concentrate on interests for which there has earlier been no time. Others view the prospect with dread, wondering how they will fill the hours once the workplace no longer provides structure and discipline in their lives.

The fifties is often a time of tumultuous change in family life. Children who were still moving in and out of the family home a decade ago have fled the nest completely, now firmly established in their own lives. Grandchildren are putting in an appearance. Homes often have to be 're-childproofed'; child management skills have to be revived and, sometimes, relearned to take account of a new generation's theories and philosophies. For many women, husbands, so often older than wives, are suddenly at home all the time, demanding cups of tea and meals and attention from a spouse who has been largely free for years to follow her own interests and inclinations. Just as the requirements of children are receding, ageing parents may impose new demands, often more extreme both emotionally and physically than the demands of small babies.

Women often complain that they become invisible as they age and it is not only in shops and on public transport that they have reason to feel disregarded. In her book *The Beauty Myth*, Naomi Woolf asserts that women's magazines 'ignore older women or pretend they don't exist', and it is a point which is hard to deny. As anyone who is even faintly familiar with the bulk of popular women's magazines can testify, the only older women commonly featured are those such as Joan Collins who are admired almost solely for their ability to disguise the fact of their age, whether by judicious make-up or photographic retouching, or as a result of surgery. In this book, Kendra Sundquist recounts her outrage at seeing a *Women's Weekly* cover photo of Maggie Tabberer and her partner, Richard Zacchariah, with the caption, OLDER WOMAN, YOUNGER MAN – HOW DOES SHE COPE? As Kendra drily observed, given Maggie's beauty and vitality it might have been more appropriate to ask HOW DOES HE COPE?

Women in their fifties today grew up in an era when the role of traditional wife and mother was hardly questioned. For most, the twenties were when they married and coped with small children. The thirties were the years of canteen and tuckshop duty, ferrying children to school and sporting activities. The forties were taken up ministering to the needs of teenagers and launching young adult offspring into the world. Suddenly, at fifty, there is a pause and time to take stock of one's own life, to ask, who am I? what do I want?

The answers are not always easy. At fifty, it is no longer possible to blame inadequacies and deficiencies on other people. At fifty, whatever is missing in your life, *you* have left it out.

But, as the women in this book demonstrate beyond any doubt, any negatives can be turned into positives. The fifties is a time to branch out in new directions, conscious that although decades spent ministering to the needs of others may have submerged personal happiness, now is the time to make up some lost ground. It is not 'too late'. Our years of maturity are barely half-way gone and there is no reason why the coming decades cannot be exciting and fulfilling and a time of opportunity to fit the missing pieces in the jigsaw of our life experience.

The fifties is a time when we find our own voice, and our own autonomy and we are not any longer defined by our relationship to others. The fifties is a time when we move from survival to mastery, from being swept solely by the currents of other people's demands and expectations to taking responsibility for our own destiny, acting for ourselves rather than simply reacting to others.

Women in their fifties today have seen more change in their lifetime than any previous generation. They have experienced twenty-five years of feminist thought. They have seen it become possible for women to control their own fertility. They have lived through the demand for equal rights in the workplace, and the enshrining of principles of equal opportunity in legislation. They have seen maternity leave become integral to conditions of employment. They have been part of the fight for the recognition that women are entitled not to have unwelcome sexual attention foisted on them. They have been at the beginning of the demand for a sharing of domestic and child-rearing burdens. They have gone from an era when virginity before marriage was assumed to see living together outside marriage become commonplace.

Now, with half a century of life behind them, fiftysomething women are beginning to redefine the parameters of age. Hormone replacement therapy has lessened and even removed most of the difficulties of menopause and so they no longer dread its discomforts or see it as a signal of inevitable physical decline.

Feminism has taught them that they are entitled to be taken account of and have their needs considered and so they are unlikely to accept being rendered invisible. The lifting of sexual taboos has taught them that they are entitled to be sensuous and to expect sexual pleasure and so they are unlikely to accept being rendered sexually obsolete. Feminism has taught them that they are entitled to intellectual satisfaction and achievement and so they are unlikely to accept being sidelined in the world of work until they are ready. Changing attitudes have enabled them to realise that although they value home and family they are entitled to other sources of satisfaction too and so they are unlikely to define their identity solely as the derivative one of grandmother becoming, in a re-run of earlier years, merely a surrogate parent, a baby-sitter and potty-trainer to a new generation while their daughters go off to be part of the corporate battle.

This book set out to find out from nine women between fifty and sixty what this time of their life means to them. What are the myths and what are the realities? Are there common features that can usefully be passed on to those coming up behind? What were their life experiences in their younger years? What are their main motivating forces now? Where is the feminist movement today? Should it now be turning its attention to older women? Are older women being overlooked by their younger sisters, just as they have been overlooked by society in general? What about sexuality — does it decline? What about menopause — are the difficulties real or imagined? How do they view the future? Is the approach of old age a matter for apprehension? What about one's inner self, one's creative and spiritual being? What is success? Do we redefine it? Should we redefine it?

The women have a wide variety of backgrounds and experiences. Some are well known and have achieved much in the public arena. Some are completely unknown outside their own circle of family and friends. Some, like Eve Mahlab, Wendy McCarthy and Quentin Bryce, combined a career with family obligations from the very first. Some, like Jeannette McHugh and Helen Leonard, fulfilled a traditional role for most of their adult life and only moved outside that role much later, sometimes by choice, sometimes by force of circumstance. Some, like Anne Ferguson, pursued a career but only now find themselves free to let their creativity have full rein without the constant distractions of family. Some, like Kendra Sundquist and Sara Henderson are blazing with energy and accomplishment, determined to achieve as much as they can after years of suppressing their own talents and ambitions. Some, like Nene King, have opted out of super-achievement, conscious that the cost to personal life and close relationships is too high. Some have had extraordinary sadness, even tragedy, to cope with. Some are financially secure as they face a winding down of their earning life and some are not. Some are in a long-standing and stable relationship, some are confronting life alone.

Whatever their story and their personal circumstances, some things are common to all the women. There was no one who did not express a sense of liberation, of glowing self-confidence, of an awareness, often only recently realised, that they could achieve more than they had ever imagined. They have a sense of energy and vitality and competency greater than at any previous stage in their lives. They report a calmness, a wisdom and a tolerance unknown in their youth. They have left confusion, insecurity and emotional turmoil behind and found in their place a sense of direction, confidence and a certain toughness. They have come to care more about how they feel than about what people think. They know what they want and how to pursue it.

It was interesting, and salutary, to take note of Eve Mahlab's cautionary note that the fifties are not fabulous for many women and that this book would do women a disservice if it implied that all in the middle-aged garden was wonderful. Of course it is not and there are hurdles and difficulties to be overcome at this age just as at any age. But what became clear as the interviews progressed was that whatever the individual circumstances of these women, even if they have little money and indifferent health, even if they are alone, without the emotional and physical support of a partner, there is nevertheless a sense of optimism about the future, a feeling of self-worth, of inner contentment and an ability to cope with whatever lies ahead.

For me, the opportunity to compile this book has been an enormous privilege. The women shared their lives with me with a generosity I found touching and moving and for which I owe them all a tremendous debt of gratitude. They were open and honest and direct. Often their voices broke with emotion as they recalled painful events in the past. But at no stage did they resile from the task at hand. They knew that their experiences might help other women, enable other women to confront and overcome difficulties and sadnesses in their lives, encourage them to grasp nettles and have the courage to achieve, make their path a little easier, and this was what they wanted above all else to do. They are indeed 'fabulous fifties' and they are all, each and every one of them, magnificent role models for the rest of us.

JAN BOWEN

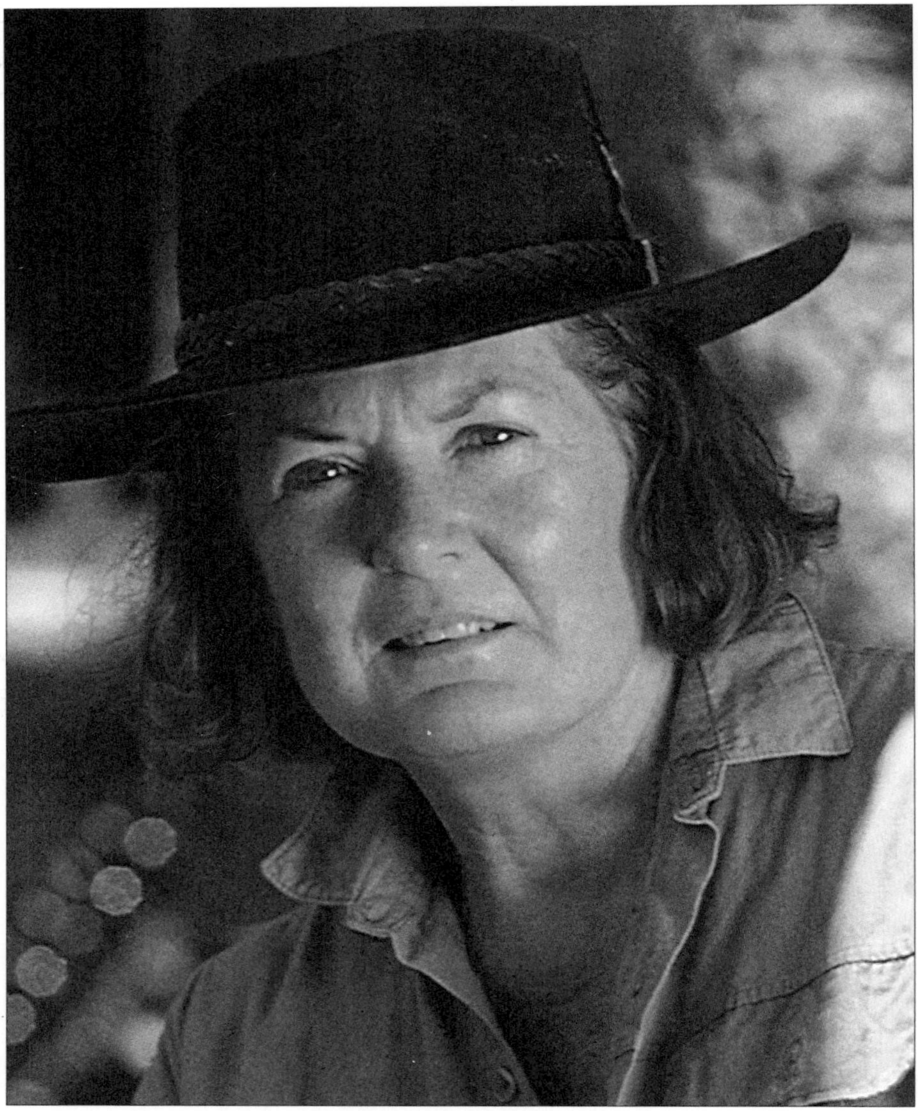

*The last eight years have been the most incredible in my life
and I think it took fifty years of experience to have been able to handle what I have had to
handle. I don't think I would have been capable of it at thirty; maybe at forty I might
have been half-way capable.*

Sara Henderson

A mere five years ago, virtually no one had ever heard of Sara Henderson. Today, there must be few people in Australia who do not know who she is. Sara first sprang to national prominence when she won the Businesswoman of the Year Award in 1991. She had been nominated by her eldest daughter, Murray Lee, and not only was she not a corporate high-flyer in the conventional sense, the entire nation was captivated by the story of how three women — Sara and two of her daughters — had pulled their remote cattle station home back from the brink of the bankruptcy into which they were catapulted after the death of Charles Henderson, in that most extreme of macho environments, the outback Northern Territory.

Following the award, Sara's rapidly commissioned autobiography, *From Strength to Strength*, chronicling her life with Charles, her American-born, swashbuckling, philandering spouse, became an instant best seller. If she had set out to write a novel, she could not have done much better. A great love affair, pirates, colourful overseas settings, quintessential Australia, crocodile wrestling, travel, hardship, beating the odds, triumph of womanhood, it was all there. But in this case, it had the added appeal of being true. Australia loved it — and Sara became an overnight celebrity.

If anyone fitted the concept of a 'fabulous fifty' it was Sara and it was with some anticipation as well as curiosity that I arranged to meet her. She is quite different from expectations. Prior to our meeting for this book, I had taken the opportunity to attend an 'authors evening' at my local library at which she was guest of honour as part of the promotion for her second book, *The Strength in Us All*. Her photo is on the cover of both books, and I tried to identify her in the small, obviously 'official' group. It seemed that she had not yet arrived as there was no one amongst the gathering who matched the cover photos. I simply did not recognise the elegantly dressed woman with the soft, waving auburn hair, standing diffidently to one side, as being the same person as the somewhat brawny, jeans-clad, Akubra-hatted image on the dust jackets of her books.

For our meeting, we had decided that my home was a better option than the impersonality of a hotel room or publisher's office and we fixed a time in the early afternoon. Sara arrived laden with parcels. She had been on a shopping spree in preparation for a forthcoming trip to England where her books were about to be published, and was bubbling over with delight at the (clearly all too rare) excuse it provided to indulge her penchant for feminine clothes.

Her air of elegant restraint was reinforced at this second meeting and I remembered how I had been struck, on reading her books, by one account of an incident where she had insisted on serving tea, in that rough outback setting, in fine bone-china cups. Now the picture was fitting together.

I found Sara to be a woman of immense charm. She is reserved and, one suspects, slightly shy but nevertheless totally straightforward and direct. Still clearly bemused by her sudden fame, she seems to handle it all with calm assurance.

Strength is a concept that looms large in Sara's life. Both her books have 'strength' as part of the title and it was the first thing she talked about in our chat. One can understand why. For a born and bred city girl, those first years on Bullo Station with no running water, no power and a tin shed for a home, must have tested her endurance to its fullest extent. And even when living conditions became easier the sheer difficulty of life in the Outback, not to mention the particular problems generated by her spouse, ensured that strength was needed in abundance. She would never have survived without it.

Whilst Sara's life could never be regarded as conventional, the role she played within the family was surely so. Until she turned fifty, she was a wife and mother in the same way as so many women of her generation, without any real identity apart from that. In essence, her husband called the shots and she supported him. She was the nurturer and the carer of the children and he was the grandiloquent adventurer, leading them into hair-raising and often downright dangerous situations, seemingly assuming that all responsibility for their wellbeing rested on her shoulders. For years she tolerated his infidelities, believing that keeping the family intact was all-important.

Sara's life in her fifties has taken off in a way that most of us could never comprehend. She is not only running an outback cattle station, she is in constant demand on the motivational speaking circuit. She now spends most of her time travelling the length and breadth of Australia and, increasingly, the world. She is so busy that when I tried to make a follow-up appointment we could not find a mutually convenient time for more than six months.

But although the details of her life are different, the fundamentals are the same. As she says, Charles died when she turned fifty and then she was free to be herself. But she was becoming herself anyway. As so many women say, the advent of the fifties is the time when they find themselves, when they have the confidence to live life as they want to, free from the restrictions and restraints of earlier years, whether self-imposed or imposed from outside. Sara Henderson is no different.

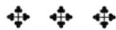

I think you look back and analyse your life as you get older. I look back over my life and the older you get, you philosophise a lot more. I think strength builds as you go, I really believe that. A lot of people aren't tested so they never find the inner strength, but if you are tested a lot, you keep finding more and more and it develops and grows. Some people are tested and they think, no, this is too much, I am not going to do it, and they go away, so they don't know if they have the strength.

I think I have had an unusual life because I married a very unusual man and I really wasn't me until I didn't have him. I think a lot of women have gone through that. They didn't discover themselves until they either lost their husband or left their husband if they had, as I had, a most domineering husband who didn't allow me to be me. I had to be for him, so I really didn't find myself until the last eight years.

I think they were there, the confidence and the strength were there, because to endure Charlie they had to be, but I didn't know they were there. There was so much pandemonium and panic in my life and I was always running behind him, always caught in the slipstream of his volatile life. I didn't have a life, I lived out of his, even though I think just surviving him I had strength.

I think I was coming into my own when he died. I was growing stronger and stronger and as I was growing older I was losing the complete awe that I had for him. As a young woman, I just adored the ground he walked on. As I got older — you never know when you get to these stages — but suddenly one day I thought, Sara, you have been had! So I started to analyse the situation and I think as I grew, I had less awe for him and I started to develop me.

I would have to say that the most striking thing about being in your fifties is confidence. I have found a confidence that I didn't think I had and I can handle things now without thinking, whereas in the earlier times I would have been terrified.

My challenges started at the age of fifty. Charlie died when I turned fifty. The last eight years have been the most incredible in my life and I think it took fifty years of experience to have been able to handle what I have had to handle. I don't think I would have been capable of it at thirty; maybe at forty I might have been half-way capable.

I find the interesting thing is that the mind doesn't age. It really doesn't. Although it depends on the person. I think how you see the world depends on your health, and what you eat, and how you live life, and your values. I am fifty, I have nearly finished my fifties, but I don't feel it.

Feminism came into vogue when we had no communication at Bullo. The last I read or heard about feminism was burning bras and the other classic remark was 'ban labour pains'. With those two statements I thought, if that is feminism I want nothing to do with it. I think it has certainly grown and evolved and I totally agree with issues like equal pay for equal jobs. I don't think that ability has gender and if people just repeated that to themselves quite often, there wouldn't be so many problems for women. I know it is very difficult for women in some areas of life to survive because they are up against the glass ceiling, they are up against a lot of things. At the present time, I think men are terrified of women, so we have to work through that. In my opinion, women hold the power to do anything and I don't think they should wait and sit at home complaining. They should just do it, in a very civilised, quiet manner. We raise the children so if women are complaining about the way men treat them, who have they got to blame but themselves, because they raised the men. If a boy child is to have the attitude towards women that a woman wants, all she has to do is raise the children in that way and then her sons will treat the next generation of women correctly. I think it is all in our hands. I would say to any woman who was complaining, stop complaining and change it.

I don't know when I had menopause, but apparently it has passed and that is marvellous. When Charles was ill my periods stopped and that was it. I suppose it was just the unbelievable stress and I didn't have time to think about it. The last eight years I have been fighting day and night to survive. Now I am through the hard times, menopause has gone too. I went to the doctor not long ago and he looked at my card and he said, 'Good heavens, you are fifty-eight,' and I said, 'Yes, I think so,' and he said, 'When was your menopause?' and I said, 'I don't know.' Then he said, 'Well, what about this?' and I said, 'No.' 'Hot flushes?' 'No.' He went through the whole lot and I said, 'No,' but he said, 'You are fifty-eight,' and I said, 'Please don't keep telling me that.' He gave me a couple of tests and he said I passed.

Family has always been very special to me. I grew up in a large family with four brothers, and of course in those days they wouldn't show affection towards their little sister, they would give you a cuff over the ears before they would be gentle or loving towards you; well, never loving, but if you were in danger or if someone was being a bully they would be there in an instant to back you up. Even though it wasn't admitted, the family always stuck together. I grew up that way and when I look back now I realise that I was very fortunate to have had a very happy family and a secure base.

Now with my own family, it is the same. We are friends, mother and daughters. My daughters are exceptional girls. They are very independent, they are thoughtful, they will take on anything as challenges and they are just good people.

I have always joked with my children that they were all mistakes. And they were, contraceptive mistakes, because I was not up with the methods. That really upset one of them. The other two laughed but one was quite upset and I said, 'Look, I think the world of you and once I was pregnant I would never think of not having you.' But I do think often that I'd still be deciding, should I have a child, if I'd had to decide.

I don't know why. I think it was the unknown and you hear all the horrendous stories about childbirth so that I thought, I don't like the sound of that. Also, I had always been an athlete, and in those days having your body out of shape was something that you would hide. Now women are being photographed nine months pregnant and it is not an awful thing, but in those days you went into hiding when you were pregnant. The royal family never appeared in public after four months. That is what I was raised with. As a younger woman you had the concept that your body wasn't beautiful when you were pregnant. So, being an athlete and always having a body that was toned and muscled and in shape, it frightened me that I would be out of shape. And of course I thought Charlie wouldn't love me if I was out of shape. You think in that small cell, you don't think that your husband will still think you are beautiful, and you don't find out differently until you are older. When I was about forty-eight — and by then you think you are starting to age — one night Charlie was most upset because he said that this man was making eyes at me at a particular dinner. I said, 'Good heavens, Charlie, he is twenty-five, why would he be looking at me with all these young girls around?' He said, 'Well, you look lovely,' and I realised that his eyes were fading and he couldn't see the wrinkles. To him, I was still as I was when I was twenty-five and he married me. So all these things change and I realised at that late stage in life that he probably thought I looked beautiful when I was pregnant. But when you are young you think it is horrible, or we did, because we were raised to hide ourselves in the last five months of pregnancy.

Raising three very independent daughters is probably my greatest achievement. Of course, their dad had a tremendous effect on them too. He demanded that they produce the best that they possibly could and somehow he got that across to them. I gave them standards that I thought they should live up to, so between us we set a path for them and we were lucky that they found this important enough to follow. I think raising three lovely daughters is pretty good in this day and age.

My other big achievement was saving Bullo, because when Charles died it was on the verge of bankruptcy.

I think I stayed with Charlie partly because there was an underlying sense of wanting to, but also I think it evolved out of my training. I was taught that marriage was very serious and it was something that you didn't take lightly: the vows that you made in church were for ever and you had to put the best into it. Of course, I was very much in love with him. When we separated, I think it was a combination of growing up and knowing more about life and slowly but surely losing that idol love. I idolised him and so my love grew out of that. That slowly receded and I slowly grew up. Also, the traditions that I grew up with broadened.

For me, creativity is only becoming evident now that I am getting older.

Again, Charlie was all my life; he demanded everything. I think the creativity was there because I can remember, looking back, that I would think of something and think it would be a great plot for a book. Things would go through my mind constantly. But I didn't have the time when I was married to him, to actually stop and think that I would like to try and write it.

I have been asked a lot of times if writing is cathartic for me, but it isn't really. I think I am basically practical and, as I said in the book, when I wrote the first draft it was all the clean linen and all the dirty linen was left in the cupboard. I looked at it and admitted to myself that I had gone around all the bad things and made Charlie look like he was a knight in shining armour, and he wasn't. I sat and thought, if you are going to write this book you tell it as it is. But there were lots of really deep things that I couldn't ever put in print and I wouldn't put in print because of the hurt of other people. So I decided with myself that Charlie is gone and I can't hurt him, so I will make him the scapegoat. He left me a million dollars in debt and I think I have the right to tell the world what he was like. So I did. There was no cleansing, or that this had to come out before I became me. It was easy to write. I just sat down and I wrote it. It was no great tearing of the soul.

My daughters all reacted differently. Marlee was very proud and that is the way she is. She said, 'It's great, Mum, it will be a best seller,' and I kept saying to her that she is a little biased because anything I do she says, that's it, that will be great. Bonnie and I weren't speaking at that time, so she didn't give me her opinion. Danielle, the youngest, was embarrassed. She didn't know how to handle it and when the book was about to come out she said, 'I'm not going to tell anyone you are my mother.' I said, 'That's alright. If you feel that you can't handle this and you are embarrassed by it, that's fine, but I have to do this to save Bullo. The publishers are interested in my life story so I have to tell it how it was.' When the book came out it was very popular. Danielle lives in a country town and it was especially popular in the country, and people would come up to her and say, 'I think your mother's book is absolutely wonderful.' About six months after it came out she would ring up and say, 'I have about six friends who would like you to personally sign the book.' It slowly brought her around.

I do find the prospect of my body ageing bothers me. You have to. I think I am accepting it gracefully because I don't try to dress as if I am still young. I dress comfortably and I don't wear high heels because it is much better to wear flat ones. If I go somewhere at night for dinner I will wear a higher heel, but I don't try desperately to look young, or not ridiculously young. I think that every woman has that fear of losing their looks. I don't care who it is, or if they say they don't care. They do. You have to think about it sometimes. The ABC did a movie on us when I was thirty, and I look at it and think, good heavens, what is happening? I used to hear of old movie stars watching their young films, and I now think it is very bad to look at yourself when you were young. You should just age and look at yourself as you go along.

I find now that I am very, very sensitive to everything I do in regard to my health. Health is becoming a priority because I think whether you can help it or not, you are thinking ahead and you are hoping that you will still be fit to the last minute. I have decided that I will do everything I can to make sure I am. I don't drink, I never did smoke and every bit of food I eat now I am very conscious of. I think, I am not going to eat that because it is not going to help the body. I try to eat the best food I can to make the body work. I work on the principle of an engine: if you put top-grade fuel in it and you oil it constantly and you look after it, it will go further.

I would never have a face-lift. I couldn't do that. Apart from anything else, I couldn't even bear to think of a knife cutting my face. I think your face is who you are and your face is what you have done. One of the most fascinating books I ever read was *The Picture of Dorian Gray*. It has stuck in my mind since the time I read it when I was twenty, and when you are twenty you never think about age. I could never do it. Marlee has just had a mole taken off her face and I saw the agony she went through. When I asked, 'Does it hurt that much?' she said, 'Mum, I'm in agony.' She had two stitches. These women who get their whole face pulled up, they don't look human. You can see them, they sit there, as if ... I am too much of a coward. Six weeks in hospital with black eyes. I think it is the mutilation of a human being and I couldn't do it. It is not just a face that is being cut, it is your life. Everything about it terrifies me.

I don't feel too old for anything yet. When I was growing up and when the children were young, I found that I would not do things because I kept thinking that if I hurt myself — if I injured myself or I died — there would be no one to look after the children. So I mentally stopped myself doing a lot of exciting things when I was younger because I felt I had an obligation to raise my children. But now that they are grown and they can look after themselves, I seem to be doing all these things. We are going to America in September and I am going white-water rafting. I would love to bungy jump. I was going to race in the celebrity race in the Grand Prix but because Marlee was injured, I had to drop everything and fly home. Now I feel I can do these things because I am only responsible for me now but I am not stupid, I won't do really dangerous things. Nor will I do all this crazy dancing, but that is because of the way I was trained. Mum took levels on what was ladylike and what wasn't. Bungy jumping sounds pretty crazy, but it isn't in that ladylike and unladylike sense. There are also clothes I won't wear because Mum said they are not ladylike clothes and that was instilled in my brain as a young girl. There is what you do and what you don't do. I wouldn't go to a disco dressed up like lamb and carry on. Even the other night when I won the book publishers' award everyone was drinking and celebrating and I couldn't do it because that is the way I was trained.

Whether those inhibitions are good or bad probably depends on the person. It depends on the individual because some of those inhibitions crushed a lot of people. People make out of it what they make out of it. With me, it has been good to have guide posts to live my life by. With friends I have known, it has inhibited them and made them a mouse. It depends on the parents. The way Charles raised the girls, it was getting to the point where he was too hard on them and I had to step in and fight to save them mentally because he was hounding them to the point where he could have crushed them. When the children were between about twelve and fifteen, Charlie and I fought tooth and nail all the time because I was protecting the girls. I do believe that a parent has a great responsibility in making sure that the way they are guiding the children is not a road that is impossible for the child to follow.

But standards are essential. In my opinion, what is missing today is religion, which is the base that children need. It has to be open enough for a child to be able to decide, and it can't be so that it pushes them into a mould that they can't handle. But it has to be there for them to decide on. The family is very, very important. It is a security base to work on. Morals are very important and another thing that is missing today is conscience. My mum raised us on conscience. Every time there was a situation she would ask us what our conscience told us and we would know straightaway right from wrong. Not always, but a good percentage of the time, as we were growing up. She would always say to us, 'Ask your conscience and if you don't have an answer, ask us and we will tell you what is right and wrong.' I think conscience is missing today.

The children of Dr Spock were a generation of rebels because they weren't controlled in any way. It went too far. The Victorian upbringing was too far the other way. There has to be a middle path. There are children brought up on that middle path, in the last generation, this generation, and they are very wholesome and polite and intelligent and I have met a lot of them. Yet there are others that are totally the other way. You have a percentage of every type in a generation. It is up to individual parents to judge their individual child and of course unfortunately there are a lot of parents lacking in ability to do that. For a majority of the population, the parents didn't have the education to foresee what they were guiding their children into.

A spiritual life was and still is very important to me. Charlie made, I think, a very profound statement when he said man is basically a religious animal. I agree with him, because you find that if people have no religion to follow they inevitably follow something, whether it is Nazism or the Ku-Klux-Klan or cults or Satan. People have to look up to something, they have to admire something. God is the best one, but God has lost His lustre at present only because of the Church. Although not for me. I still follow Him. I don't follow Him through the Church, though. The churches have lost their way. They have had power for so long and power is a fascinating thing. If people have power they sometimes lose the plot because the power takes them over. I feel the churches had unchallenged power for too long. You would not have believed thirty years ago that people would be asking if Jesus existed. Thirty years ago, you just believed it wholeheartedly. The churches have to re-shape themselves for the people to follow them again. The older generation followed because it was what we were taught, but the young people are saying, 'But I want to know,' and the Church now has to find the answers.

But to follow God between just yourself and God is very easy and very fulfilling. In the Outback I go and look at the heavens and you know straightaway that there has to be something better than you, because who could have created anything as beautiful as the sky?

I talk straight to Him and it gives me a great feeling of satisfaction even if I tell Him off, which I do. I see it as a direct conversation. I don't believe that on one hand in the Bible He says, don't do this or I will turn you into stone, and on the other hand you can do anything and get down on your knees and apologise and it is all forgotten. That doesn't correlate for me, so I just talk to Him and when I think things are wrong, I tell Him so. He has never hit me with a bolt of lightning, and I tell Him off quite often. I tell Him the world is in a mess and if He created us and put us here for a purpose, then His experiment is a bit off line. He should be a bit more forgiving and tender with the people He hasn't given everything to, like intelligence and the power to direct their lives. He should be looking after them. The person who has power and money and can direct their own life, then He doesn't have to look after them as much. I tell Him this quite often and He hasn't hit me with lightning as yet. That is the way I look at religion, it is very practical.

I don't worry too much about the future, even though I live where I do, so far from anywhere, because as we are developing the property, it becomes a more attractive place to be. If I went out there now, approaching sixty, as I did when I was twenty-eight, I couldn't do what I did, but each year it gets more humanised and it is a very lovely place to live now. I suppose when I am eighty or ninety it might be a problem but with your own plane and town a couple of hours away ... and in another thirty years it will probably be populated.

It would be a hard place to be if one was physically frail but I don't think I will ever be physically frail. I have never been frail, so I think I have the physical stamina, so long as I never get ill, to endure out there. You see a lot of people that are seventy-five and eighty still riding horses and rounding up cattle so, if God is willing, I will be out there until I am about eighty. But I love the sea, so if I had to I could retire to somewhere by the sea where it is quiet.

I think getting older is much easier for women than men. Women can still do things, especially sexually. I think that shows with the men because the older they get the younger the women they chase. The men in my age group are all looking at thirty-year-olds because they are hanging on to youth and as they get older their performance potential goes down and they are terrified. I wouldn't like to be a man for anything. Women, I think, have it much easier.

Friends are essential in your life, along with your family. I think the two assets of a long life are family and friends. I don't have a lot of women friends, because of where I live, but the ones that I have I treasure. My sister is my greatest friend and I have a few school friends that are still very close. Even though we don't see each other so often there is a lot of telephone communication. Murray Lee is one of my closest friends because we worked through eight years together and we have both lost our husbands in that time so the bond I have with her is brilliant. Both of my daughters are also my friends. One of my sisters-in-law is very close and a couple of my nieces, along with different friends I have made along the way. I have met a lot of people in the last eight years which is fascinating and some are great friends now. Of course, when we went to the station it was very difficult to see friends because we were so isolated for the first ten or eleven years. But I have friends in America who go back thirty years, since before I went to Bullo, also in Hong Kong and now that things are happening with my book in England, I am travelling more, so I can renew friendships that have been there all those years.

I would like to think that I would have another relationship in my life. It would be different, though. You can never have that young love that you had before, and I am changed, so I look at men in a totally different way now. But I would love to meet a nice man.

I love to write, so if I can keep writing I would find that very beneficial. The station is a full-time occupation so if I can run the station and write I think I will have a great life. If I could add a nice man, then I would have paradise. I don't hold much hope for meeting the man because I get the impression that men go around me like they are walking on eggs. Because of the publicity I've received, men seem to think that I am a bit invincible so they don't want anything to do with me. They think, I am not going to take her out, she has done too much. I haven't really done anything, but the media have built it up.

All the reporters keep asking, 'Are you going to get married again, are you going out with men?' You can't just say, 'Well, they don't ask me,' because you think maybe there is something wrong or you are too old. So I thought this year I would slim down and get into shape again and if they still don't ask me, then I know I have a problem.

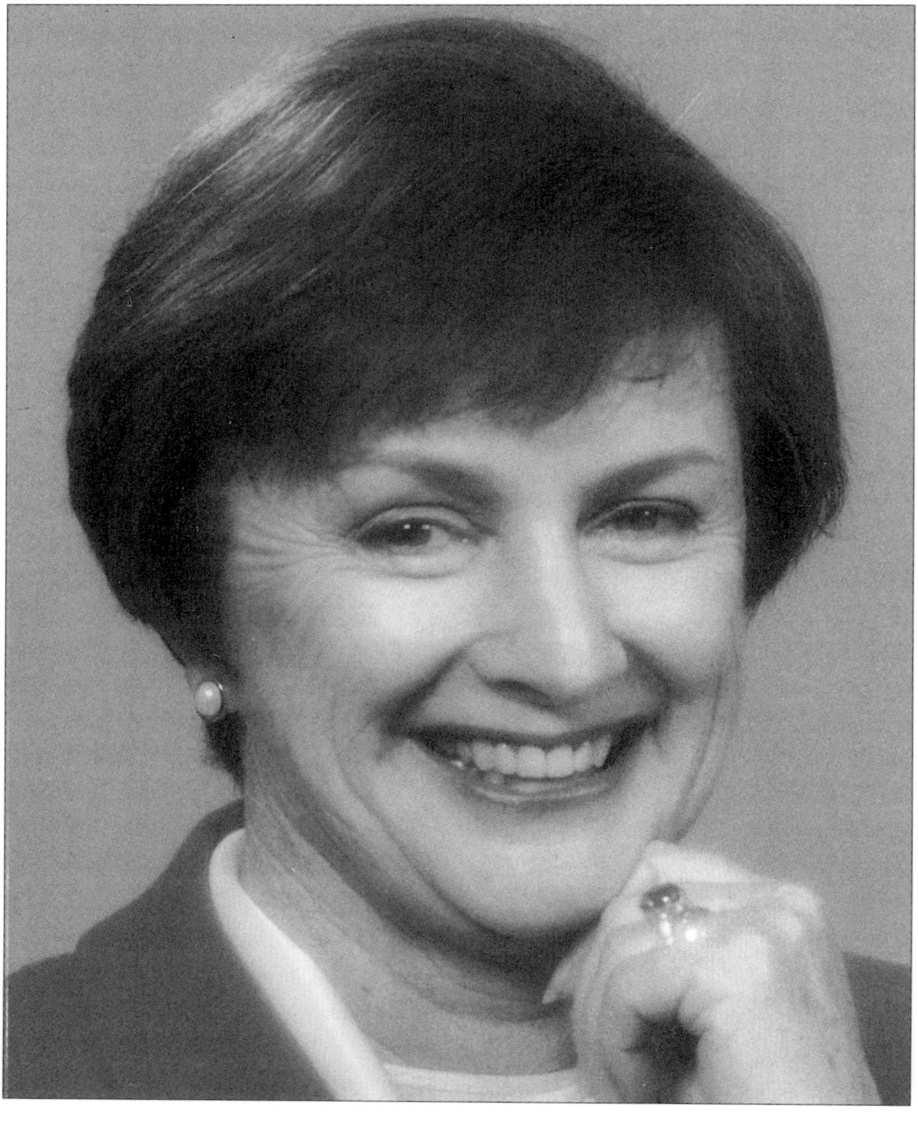

The fifties are so liberating. I've done with all the expectations, I have been a mother, I'm a wife, I've done the working. I've learned about the conflict of trying to keep all those balls up in the air and suddenly there is time to be me.

Wendy McCarthy

A career change, a move from suburbia to a trendy inner-city pad and a short, chic, Titian-tinted hairdo; at fifty-three, Wendy McCarthy has no intention of allowing comfortable familiarity to take the edge off her need for new challenges

'Taking life more quietly' isn't in Wendy's lexicon. Having gone straight from the airport to work that morning after a trip interstate, our meeting at her home at the end of the day was punctuated by several phone calls, the need to display some motherly concern (and cash) to a son recovering from a recent illness but now well enough to venture forth for the evening, and the arrival of a dinner guest. Each interruption was dealt with calmly and efficiently and our chat resumed as if she had done no more than draw a necessary breath.

Efficiency shines out of Wendy. An attractive woman, elegantly dressed in a businesslike black suit and matching shoes enlivened by a procession of gold animals encircling the just-raised heels, every movement seems to have a purpose. Even her speech is quick and precise. This is a person who makes every moment count.

Wendy's home reflects her taste. Part of a completely renovated erstwhile warehouse, in one of the earliest parts of Sydney to be settled, the two-storey apartment envelops its occupants with curving banisters, mellow, polished floors, scattered rugs and an interesting collection of pictures on the walls. Expressing irritation that a striking ikebana flower arrangement had wilted during her absence, despite her son's inhabitancy, she made the wry observation that she supposed it would be a bit too much to expect him to notice the need for fresh water, even with the training he had been exposed to. My attention was diverted from the flowers by the view through the windows, over the city, with the twin peaks of the Opera House framed between two glittering high-rises.

Wendy and her husband, Gordon, spend weekends together, alternately in the apartment or at the Berrima farm where Gordon breeds prize-winning cattle. Their weeks are spent apart, doing what each likes best. Wendy says that marriage is the perfect human relationship when the partners are each able to grow. It was a pattern that emerged constantly during the compiling of this book. Numerous people had said to me that they imagined most of the women would be 'femes sole', their personal relationships a casualty not only of the time and effort they had put into achieving their success but also of their strong feminist principles. It proved not to be the case. More of the women than not had long-lasting and happy marriages, but it became clear that a prerequisite for that was the willingness of both parties to give one another space to pursue their own interests and activities and careers, even to the extent of living in different geographical locations for much of the time if that was what it took. It also became clear that when those adjustments were able to be made (and it must have been difficult, since the convention thirty years ago when these marriages took place was so different) the rewards were immense for both sides with each partner fulfilled and happy and able to contribute immeasurably to a relationship which they valued so much more for its capacity to allow for individual growth and satisfaction.

Wendy first came to prominence in the 1970s, with her forthright approach as information and education officer of the Family Planning Association. Barely twenty years ago, it was an era when today's open discussions about sexual matters could not have been comprehended. I recall being astonished at hearing her talk on radio one day, expressing outrage that proper contraceptive advice had not been available to her when she was engaged. No one I knew at that time would have admitted to such a need in private, let alone over the national airwaves.

From 1983 until 1992 Wendy was deputy chairperson of the Australian Broadcasting Corporation. It was a time when that organisation was going through a period of tumultuous change. It was being restructured, its funding from government was constantly under threat and new buildings were planned both in Sydney and Melbourne so that the huge staff could be housed under one roof in each city instead of in the hotchpotch of buildings to date.

As a special project, she accompanied the Sydney Symphony Orchestra on tour to the United States, acting as manager for marketing, public relations and publicity, a job which involved representing the ABC at a senior level and arranging special events to promote Australia.

Concurrently with her ABC work, in 1985, Wendy was appointed general manager communications with the Australian Bicentennial Authority, planning the celebration of the nation's bicentennial year in 1988. It was a body which, perhaps not surprisingly given its nature, was dogged by accusations of extravagance and mismanagement, and it often fell to Wendy to take a public stance defending the Authority's activities, a task she fulfilled with aplomb. The eventual celebrations will be long remembered by Australians as a very special time in the life of the nation.

In 1989 she was awarded the Order of Australia for her contribution to the bicentennial celebrations, community and women's affairs.

It was at the Bicentennial Authority, Wendy says, that she discovered her management skills and, in 1990, following the winding-up of the organisation, she became the chief executive officer of the New South Wales branch of the National Trust. This was a challenge of a different kind. The National Trust was virtually insolvent and racked by political infighting, much of it played out in the nation's media, with the old guard staunchly resisting attempts to bring the organisation into the twentieth century. Eighteen months after taking up the job, Wendy had moved the organisation into credit and had persuaded the NSW government to legislate for a new Act, streamlining the board and its responsibilities and providing for the election of board members by the membership of the Trust itself instead of by government appointment. At the time, one member of the board described her as 'the kind of CEO who comes along once in a lifetime'.

At the beginning of 1994 came a major career change — to the private sector and the conservative and rarified world of the legal profession.

A city law firm invited her to become its manager, acting as chief executive officer — the first woman in Australia to fill such a role. At the same time, she is the chairperson of Visions for the Future, a travelling science and technology exhibition which showcases the best of Australia, chairperson of the Royal Hospital for Women Foundation, a director of Sydney Harbour Casino Ltd, and the Royal Australian College of Physicians Education and Research Foundation, a member of the Clean Up Australia Trust, the University of Canberra Council, and the Macquarie Graduate School of Management Advisory Board. She was also only the third woman in Australia to be invited to join Rotary.

With all that, slowing down is clearly very much in the future.

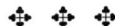

I have often thought about things that propelled me into my life and to do certain things and it is very hard to find reasons. I was the eldest daughter born to a very young mother — eighteen years of age — and a father of twenty-six. My mother came from a family of seven children and my father was one of three and they both had expectations of a traditional family life. I think that probably one of the most formative influences in my life in early times was that for four years I was an only child. I subsequently had three siblings but we were well spaced and I think that I was the centre of my parents' attention. I was certainly encouraged to achieve from the very earliest age. When I got brothers and sisters, I don't ever remember being jealous, nothing but thrilled. So, clearly, my parents had done a very good job in encouraging me to achieve and being secure in those formative years.

I think my mother grew up with me in many ways. When she was thirty-six, I was eighteen and so she confided in me a lot when I was growing up. My parents' marriage turned out to be a really difficult and unsuccessful marriage and I took a lot of responsibility in the family in terms of being my mother's confidante and accepting responsibility for the welfare of the other children. I think I probably thrived on it even then, and I was encouraged to do it. My father used to confide in me sometimes but my father had a problem with alcohol and I think that probably one of the most formative things in my life was to know that I never wanted to be as vulnerable as my mother was to the pressures that put on the family.

We went to live right out in the bush when I was seven. My father won a soldier's settlement block in a ballot. He had come from the land and for him getting back to the bush was everything. So I had a life of independence even then. I rode a bike five miles to school, or rode a horse occasionally. I was in a one-teacher school and I was always the only person in my class so, again, I tended to be given responsibility, encouraged to get on by myself. Half my time was filled in with reading books and listening to ABC radio. I didn't develop at all mathematically but I got verbal skills.

I think too, during that time when things were pretty tough, with my mother holding the family together and my father drinking quite heavily in bouts, there was a lot about wanting not to be vulnerable to the vicissitudes of things that are outside your control. Even then I think we understood that it was an illness that he couldn't control. We had some pretty hairy times but my mother worked really hard at making sure that we had standards. We were always well dressed and we were well fed and we had and were encouraged to have a certain kind of pride and style.

Living on the land in a place where there was money for a lot of the kids to go to boarding school and suddenly there wasn't money for me to go to boarding school was also important. I went into the local high school and I lived in this wonderful Anglican hostel run by a young minister and his wife who were very powerful influences in my life. First of all I got heavily into religion which started quite a long love affair — High Church Anglican. Also, I was introduced to classical music, I was introduced to a sense of my own self-esteem and, while I don't consciously remember anyone ever saying that I could do anything, I never thought I couldn't. I was always encouraged to believe I could do anything I wanted to do.

Because my family's financial position was so shaky my mother managed to get a wartime services fund to subsidise my boarding fees. So I was taught from the age of eleven when I went to high school that in order to be rewarded I had to perform. I couldn't have stayed at that school and I couldn't have stayed at an Anglican hostel because of the fees, I would have been at home doing correspondence or living with a family in the town, if I hadn't had that support. That meant my life was dependent on my report card at school and it made a big difference.

When I left school, I was the first person in our family ever to go to university. I got a few scholarships to university and everyone was totally surprised. We eventually decided that I should take the teachers college scholarship because it paid a living-away-from-home allowance. I went to New England University where I met a wonderful woman who was college principal and who totally reinforced the view that girls could do anything. She would never have used words like sexism but she just really encouraged you to get on with it.

I was only a very average university student. I worked out very early in the piece that passing was what mattered and having a good time was what mattered. That's really all I did.

My father died when I was seventeen and in early second year university and really it was a relief because it was one whole area of life that you didn't have to contend with any more. It had been miserable for him and for us for a few years. But I think then I saw how incredibly vulnerable my mother was. She had no job skills, no money and she still had an eight-year-old child to support. At least at a subliminal level I wanted to be sure that I wasn't going to be like that. My mother was extremely encouraging that I should have an education and be able to support myself.

I started my working life as a secondary school teacher and then when I was married, three years after I had started teaching, the man I married wanted to travel. So I became the first one in the family to travel. Then we lived overseas. I guess there were two things that happened in those six years. The first three years when I was teaching, I became very aware very early on that the best teachers in the school, the most professional with the greatest skills, had had to make a choice between a career or a marriage. I remember thinking how unfair it was. There were some terrific women teachers who were married and had raised families and who were working, but they never had security of tenure and, while I wasn't an activist in any way about it, I was filing it all away. I remember one of them gave me *The Feminine Mystique* to read and I knew what she was saying, not from my own experience, but I was looking at my mother and her friends and seeing how dependent they were. I don't want to denigrate their lives by saying I didn't want to be like them, because in many ways I did want to be like some of the things about them, but I didn't want that life pattern for myself. Certainly when I married Gordon I married him in the knowledge that he didn't want to be a parent for a while at least and I had made a decision that I wasn't going to be a parent until he wanted to be too. I always knew I wanted to have children. But I realised that those women, whom I grew incredibly fond of, had had to make those choices and I thought it was unjust. I could see all these men around who were enhanced by being parents and I couldn't see why women couldn't be.

When I went to live in London, one of the things that I found really remarkable was that I met all these women who never intended to have children. I started reading women like Antonia Fraser and I thought, she writes, she works as a professional author, she's married and she has six children! I saw all these middle-class British women who had au pairs and nannies and so on, and it never occurred to them that they shouldn't go back to work if that's what they wanted to do. So I began to think, well, we're all the same, how come it's so different in our culture?

Then we lived in America and I saw what we used to call the PHT syndrome — Putting Hubbie Through — women with fantastic academic qualifications who stopped to have children, or went to work so the husband could get a degree and I thought, well, I'm not interested in that. So by the time I got back here I was ready for some significant changes.

After we were married we stayed away for three years, so we became very dependent on each other in terms of sustenance and our relationship and learning to live without family or anything else. It was an incredibly liberating experience to be entirely on our own for the first three years of our marriage. Also, we both worked and we both developed a really equal relationship and I think that has been a very sustaining thing throughout my life. I am still married to Gordon after thirty years and we still give each other a lot of room to move.

I married a very unusual man who was certainly ahead of his time. When we came back to Australia, we wanted to buy a house. We didn't have a lot of money and he took the view, probably before I did, that having a baby, looking after a baby, wasn't a full-time job and if we wanted to own a house I would have to make some financial contribution to it. There were times when I resented that. On the other hand, when Sophie, our first-born, was about six months old, I found I was beginning to look around for things to do. Although I had been very actively involved in the Childbirth Education Association, which was the first major thing I had ever joined in my life, and I got involved in a resident action movement, I decided that I didn't like the feeling of being totally financially dependent on my husband. Gordon didn't like the feeling of me being totally financially dependent on him either and it just seemed to be logical that I would look for a job. So I started to look and I found it very, very hard to get a job. That made me very angry because I knew I was an extremely good teacher. Finally I got a job at a school where I worked three and a half days a week and my family, especially my mother, was extremely disapproving and really quite awful to me. My mother-in-law wasn't game enough to be really awful to me but she was extremely disapproving and people were very disapproving to Gordon. They said, can't you support your wife, what's wrong with you? He was ahead of his time in that he never felt that it was any reflection on him that I went to work. I didn't either, it used to enrage me.

During eight years of part-time work, I learned about how communities work, I got totally involved in the women's movement through abortion law reform and childbirth education and I did a lot of part-time work teaching at TAFE and various other things. I was one of the three founding members of the Women's Electoral Lobby in New South Wales. But I can still remember the day I drove down the Pacific Highway thinking, I am doing all this theoretical stuff about women, and if I go back as a teacher, which I really love, and Gordon stays as the supporter, I will end up as 'the mother' and 'the teacher' who comes home early and does all the mothering and nothing will ever change and I am not going to do it. So I started looking for a job that was different and I got a job working for Family Planning, which was just wonderful.

I was the first Education and Media information officer and that was a really liberating thing for me because I was absolutely fascinated by birthing and the human rights attached to birthing. That had started for me both in the UK and the USA. I was really interested in looking at how women were birthing there. I never heard of women having babies at home until I lived in London. When I lived in America, the women I knew used to talk about doing it with mirrors. I was never quite sure what they were doing but it seemed that they were birthing looking at mirrors. When I came back here I was very assertive about the fact that this was something that was of mega importance in my life. I was only going to do it a few times and I was going to do it under the best possible circumstances. That was the beginning for me of political activity. I hunted around until I found an obstetrician who (a) encouraged Gordon to be there and (b) encouraged me with the view that *I* was having the baby, not the doctor, and that I wanted to be as awake and aware as possible and I wanted to do natural childbirth. So in 1968 when we came back from America, I was newly pregnant and very sure that I was going to have my rights in hospital. And it all happened — Gordon was there, and everything was fine. That was the beginning for me of joining, and community and political action. It was really just a natural step.

To me, still, fertility underpins everything a woman can feel. It was certainly the cutting edge of feminism. There is no doubt in my mind that the re-defining of women's sexuality and their ability to birth or not to birth as they chose was the cutting edge of taking back power for themselves because it is something that had been taken away from them. You think about how doctors would say, here's your baby, as though they had done it. That used to make me really angry. Birthing for me was just a fantastic experience. The other day my children asked me if there is anything in my life that I regret and I said, yes, that I didn't have more children. I did love the whole thing about it. I loved that sense, that essence, of expressing yourself and being able to control your own sexuality and your own reproductive life.

So for me it was the most wonderful thing to be involved with childbirth education. I saw abortion as just the flip side of childbirth education. That is what had to be there if other things didn't work for you, it was part of the choice process. To lobby for that and to work in Family Planning was incredibly rewarding. When I joined Family Planning it was the first time it was government funded. I had to persuade the government to keep on funding it so, from 1975 to 1984, which was the decade for women, I was totally involved in women's politics. I made eleven films, I had a radio program, I had a magazine column on sexuality, I was the sex advisor to *Cleo* for nine years and also to the *Sunday Mirror*. I had that ability to be up front.

I still think that the revolution in contraception was one of the most powerful changes in how women saw themselves. It gave them that sense of control. It was probably quite hard at times for my family for me to be so outspoken on those issues but I never ever thought for one minute that it was wrong.

I look back and I think that the 1970s was the decade of consciousness-raising and I am really glad I was there doing it. The 1980s was the time when you started to implement and put down the base. The 1990s is the time to start thinking about where to next. I am glad I am in my fifties because I feel freer than I ever have in my life. I am virtually finished raising the children. There is not much I can do except be their confidante and friend now. I think that's important but it is not like I am responsible on a daily basis for them. I have moved my living so that Gordon and I can live more as we were before we were parents and try and rationalise the way in which we live. I feel free to be able to eat, manage my life, do what I want to do when I want to do it. It's a freedom underpinned by hormone replacement therapy, tubal ligation, having had a successful family-planning cycle for my life, and my own income, economic independence. It's something that most women of my age, or ten years older than me, wouldn't have dreamed of.

I guess the other fantastic thing for me about being fifty is that I can see there are heaps of opportunities for being creative for women behind me and I am glad about that.

Now I am at the cutting edge of the way society views older women. Even though I'm tired and I think to myself, I wish I didn't have to go to work because I am sick of working, then I think, look, Wendy, you are going to live until you are eighty: that's thirty years from now, and if you look back thirty years to when you were twenty, you can't afford to have the sort of lifestyle that you might want to have. You can't afford to think of yourself as a kept woman, because you are not, so you have to find ways to accommodate your needs in terms of your income and your lifestyle and it probably has to be a new format.

The other thing is that I want to be recognised as still being a contributor with the wisdom and experience that I have acquired over these thirty years in the same way as I see quite able men — as well as quite dysfunctional men — being rewarded in their sixties with board appointments and elder statesmen privileges. I think that I have made my contribution to this society, in this country, with a whole lot of other women, and I want us to be there too. I'm not giving it up now. I think if there is one hundred per cent of power available in the world I want my gender to have fifty per cent. It ought to be fifty-one per cent but I'll settle for fifty. As we get older we outlive the men so it is even more inequitable what's happening. Women over fifty are consigned to the slag heap but here they are living these long lives and the men, whose numbers are decreasing, are represented way out of proportion in all corporate governances, legislatures and so on in terms of making decisions about the way we live in the next thirty years of our lives. Well, I'm not about to put up with that so I am going to be an outrageous old woman.

In terms of women in their fifties grouping together to achieve their aims, the Older Women's Network is a very strong network, but those women are probably quite a lot older, in their seventies. I think that women in their fifties are not going to group together with that kind of a title because they don't see themselves as older. For women, being in their fifties now is like being forty used to be and I think that we are not going to group in that way. We group in other ways. We group in terms of networking about work, we group in terms of social life.

I find that there are a lot of my peer group who are making the decision that I have just made, to leave suburbia and move into the inner city because that's where the energy and the life pattern reside. That's where you can plan for the next stage of your life, to be able to walk everywhere, and do all the things that you want to that are different, and you say, a discrete part of my life raising the children in the suburbs is over. I think you will find really interesting women's activity. Already I know that older women are battling about superannuation, about discrimination, about age of retirement. I think there is a strong network, there is still the Women's Electoral Lobby network and then there are particular interest groups, such as the Older Women's Network and Grey Power, the pensioner movement. I know quite a bit about what they do, most of them tell me, and there are more of those groups than there ever were. Also, as more women of my age leave the full-time workforce with some financial security, I think we will start to have an impact in the way we buy housing, residential property and so on.

I don't think we know how the impact will occur, but I am sure it's going to happen. There is a critical mass of educated women coming through and that is what will change things because this group of women is used to having attention paid to it. If you look around now at women, even in their sixties and seventies, whom you notice, they tend to be very glamorous and well groomed, very articulate, very well off and that's why they're visible. There are a very few of them in powerful positions. One is Liz Kirkby [leader of the New South Wales Democrats], who's an interesting woman. She is always immaculately groomed, she looks sensational, she's outspoken, she's a whole new role model for people. We are just beginning to find more of those women around. If they start to penetrate the boards, which is going to be one of the hardest things to do, and they start to get those sorts of profiles in business, you will find they're carving whole new areas for themselves. I just don't think most of the women I know in that position are going to drop out of life.

I think menopause is still an individual thing and what you want most of all to encourage is the view that you are probably entering a different sexual phase of your life. The most interesting thing about it is that you are not driven by sex in quite the same way. It's that much more relaxed. That's certainly the thing that I enjoy and I didn't really realise it was happening to me until I read Germaine Greer's book on ageing and she said that suddenly you weren't following it around, it was with you when you chose, there was a kind of peacefulness about it, and that was really the breakthrough in ageing. I think that's right. I know women who are sexually active well into their seventies and I certainly hope that I am going to be. But there's a lot of peace about it and pleasure — it wasn't as peaceful even in your forties as it is in your fifties. If women adopted that view and just relaxed a bit about it — and that's certainly where new information can help, because there are creams and pessaries and hormones if you want to take them, and all sorts of other options — you are probably going to have a better sex life in your fifties than you might have had in your forties.

I am quite comfortable with hormone replacement therapy. I have watched it very carefully over the years. Although I never take very much notice of doctors who don't use things themselves, so maybe I select doctors who take hormone replacement therapy. I certainly go to women doctors to talk about my sex life or reproductive needs. In the Family Planning world, most of the women I know are using hormone replacement therapy.

The only sense of physical ageing that really bothers me is when I feel I am losing strength in my body or the ability to do things that I like to do and I can't transfer on to other things. For example, I have always liked riding horses and I fell off a horse and I have lost my nerve a bit. I don't want to be hurt that much again, so I think I have decided I am never going to ride a horse again. I might, but it will have to be a rocking-chair horse. I wish that hadn't happened because it has made me a bit timid. I don't think my body is as good at physical activity as it used to be, although I swim a lot, as I always have, I do aquaerobics, I exercise and I walk a lot. The things that I really like to do are the things that are appropriate for keeping you fit and healthy.

In terms of my face and my body, I suppose I have just accepted that gravity is moving downwards. None of this bothers me too much now. I have a GP who says every now and then, 'Are you sure you don't want to have a face-lift?' and I say, 'Well, you know...' and I put up my hands and pull my skin up and I can see things that I would like to change, but not enough to have a face-lift.

I don't know if I would ever have a face-lift. I don't think I would because I hate needles and I hate knives. I have just had a mole cut off my nose and I had twelve stitches and a black eye and a bruised face for a week. I hated that such a lot, and that's just about nothing compared with a face-lift, so I don't think I could ever do it. But I look at people who are physically aged and physically feeble and I don't want to be there for a long time.

I have friends who have had a face-lift because they want to continue in the workforce, and I have friends who have done it because of pressure from their husbands, and I have friends who have done it because they have been very, very wrinkled, and they've hated it. I don't mind if other people do. I don't have any strong feelings about that, I think that's totally their choice.

When I reached my fifties, I really wanted to make a significant change in my life about how I earned my living, what my professional skills were and how they developed. I couldn't see how I could do that unless I stopped doing the kinds of things that I was doing. So when I was offered a job to run a legal practice, which is quite different from anything I have ever done, I saw it as an interesting opportunity. Not necessarily for ever, but I never look at things as though they are for ever. I look at things in terms of what needs to be done and what I can do about it and then I tend to think it's time to move on and find something else to do. It has been a really tough six months but there's a bit of harmony coming into it now. It has catapulted me into a commercial world of professional services which is a work experience I haven't had. I am also a lot freer than when I was owned by an organisation and could really only speak publicly on its behalf in order to be effective. I wasn't gagged but I felt when I was at the National Trust that it was not a good idea for me to use up my media-allotted space by yapping on about a whole range of other things, that it was better for me to use that space for the Trust. I found that a bit constraining and here I feel totally free. That's a really nice feeling and I don't ever want to work again where I don't feel totally free.

The fifties are so liberating. I've done with all the expectations. I have been a mother, I'm a wife, I've done the working. I've learned about the conflict of trying to keep all those balls up in the air and suddenly there is time to be me. I am going off to an ASEAN Women's Conference in Singapore the week after next. Once I would never have dreamed of spending my own money on doing that. I would have thought about the money we needed in the house or all the sorts of expenses that line up with children. Now I don't have to take the responsibility for those things in the same way any more. I can do a few of the things that I want to do for myself. There is this marvellous sense of freedom.

I think that men probably don't feel that freedom until they leave work. I think their working life is just so tied to their view of themselves and supporting their families and doing all those things that I don't think they really understand what it is to be free until they retire. Then many of them find themselves trapped because they have no definition, they haven't grown up as individual people, they have just been workers. I think it is very different for men. Even women who haven't been in the paid workforce but whose children have left home, once they come to terms with that and develop their own lives, they too feel that sense of freedom. A lot of them resent it when the men hang about the house when they retire.

Families are just as important for women as they get older but we don't have to own them. We just enjoy them and we are not totally identified by them. For men, many of them haven't had that closeness and that identification and suddenly they see the family disappearing. They feel really anxious and now that's all they really care about. It can be a very disappointing time for them because by that time, if they haven't been around, most of their kids aren't that interested in them and they find that very hurtful and very disappointing. I have seen many men like that. They want to go and re-create the whole scene, build the big house and everyone to come back there and do their stuff, and the kids say, sorry, you weren't there for twenty years, not interested. Also, men often have a fantasy view of the family when they haven't been involved day by day.

The other thing is that women get more radical with age. They are more willing to take risks, they have that sense of freedom. You see women turning fifty, walking out the door of a marriage or a relationship saying, been there, done that, I'd rather live on my own, I don't have too many hard feelings but, really, that's it. I find that really interesting. I have seen a lot of people do that. They just want to carve their own bit of space and their own time.

Religion hasn't been really important in my life from the age of about eighteen on. I'm not sure whether I was in love with religion then or whether I was in love with pageantry and ritual. It was a very attractive package at the time. It was very nourishing and affirming but it hasn't been since then. My spiritual life is not connected to a religion. It's a life of reading and thinking and wondering about things but it is not connected in any way with organised religion.

My most creative years were undoubtedly in my late thirties and forties. That was my most creative period in my life so far. I don't think I'll get another one of those until I give up full-time work. I think I am on the threshold of another one. I don't want to work full-time in the long term so I have got to re-arrange my working life over the next five years. I would like to do some more writing, which I haven't done for ten years, and that's what I think will kick me off into my next creative phase.

I have got a couple of books in my head that I have been thinking about. I have been plodding away for a while and I just need the space and the time. I don't think that I have the energy any longer to go to work all day and write books all night. I did that in my thirties and forties. The family all used to go to bed at eight o'clock so I would start then. But it's too much now.

Apart from very short skirts, I can't say that there is anything that I feel too old for, but there are times when I think, I'm past that. It might be a film, it might be a concert, it might be a behaviour, but suddenly I just think, I'm past that, and I'm old enough now not to pretend. I don't have to pretend that I like it any more. That's very liberating too. I can just do what I want to do.

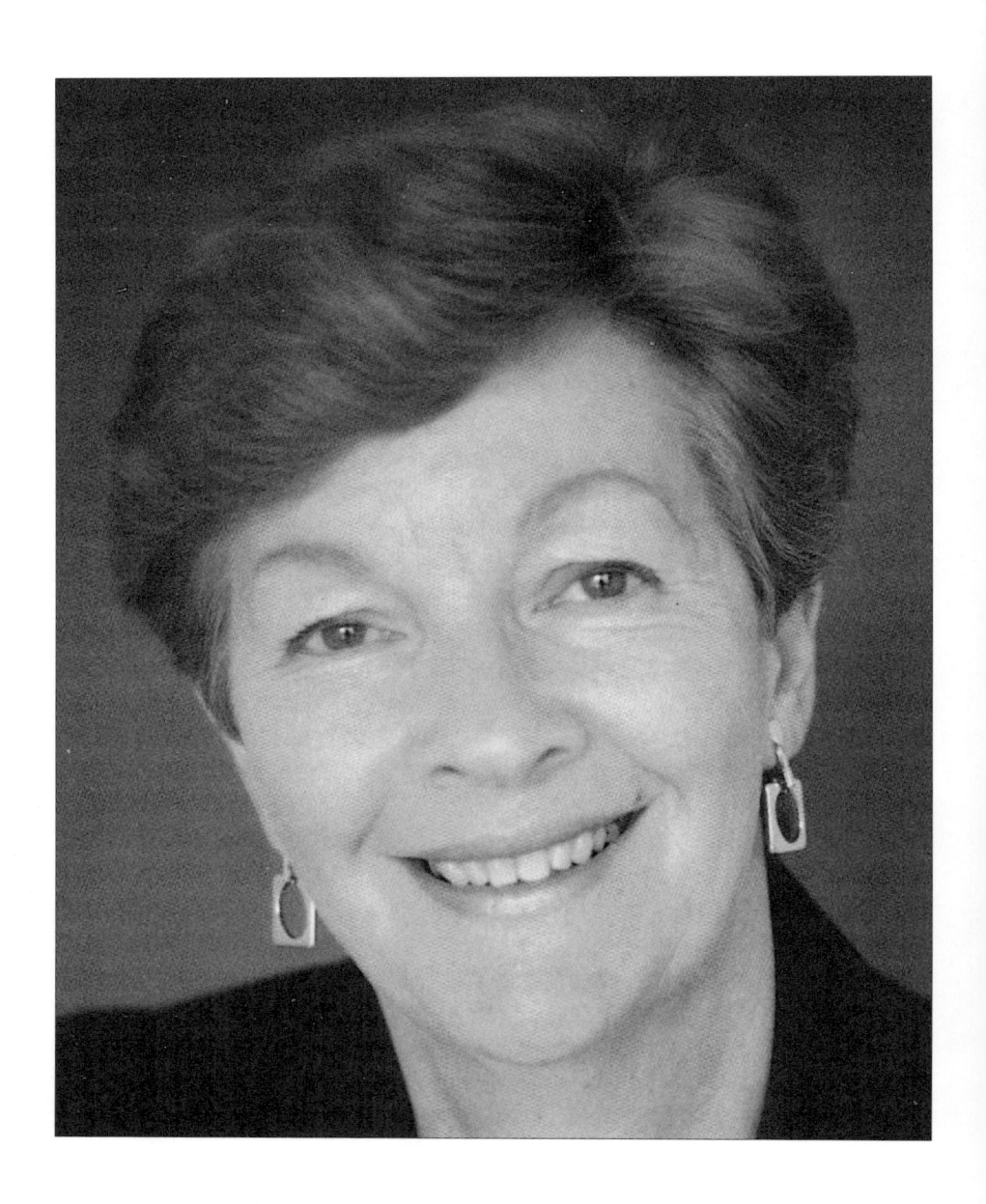

I feel I can do anything, absolutely anything. Nothing fazes me, I am not frightened any more of anything. I have a strength within myself that I didn't feel before when I felt I needed to be protected by a man.

❖ ❖ ❖

Kendra Sundquist

Kendra Sundquist had chosen to come to my home for our meeting and punctually at the nominated time I responded to the doorbell to find a smiling woman with hand outstretched, radiating warmth and instantly reinforcing the impression of friendliness I had been struck by when I telephoned to make the appointment.

As we took a little time to get to know one another, I noticed that her smart but understated skirt, blouse and blazer were enlivened by an elegant silver bracelet and earrings. With her fine, unlined skin and fashionably short hair she looked crisp and confident and well in control of her life. As we talked in more depth, her direct, calm gaze made it difficult to imagine that a few short years ago, she had thought her life might not be worth living.

I became aware of Kendra after reading an article about her in one of the Sunday newspapers. As director of education with Family Planning Australia, she had recently conducted a workshop entitled 'Mid-life: Crisis or Creativity' at a conference on sexuality. Her views on sexuality, especially as it is manifested in mature women, and her more general injunction that 'It is up to us what kind of mid-life we have. We have a choice' seemed to make her a perfect candidate for inclusion in this book.

I had no idea that Kendra's own story would prove so compelling and inspiring.

Until she was in her mid-forties, Kendra's life followed the pattern of millions of Australian women. A typical middle-class childhood in suburban Melbourne, a few years' nursing, marriage in her early twenties, two children, a bit of part-time work to enable the children to go to private schools and generally provide some pin-money — it could have been the story of virtually anyone of her generation. She fully expected that it would continue that way. As she said, 'When I was eighteen, I imagined that by this stage I would be happily at home with my husband, just pottering about in the garden.' For Kendra, her home was the focus of her life. Not having grown up in affluent circumstances, she regarded the fact that she and her husband were finally able to acquire a nice home on Sydney's North Shore as the stuff that dreams were made of and caring for her home and family was her raison d'être.

When she was forty-five, because of a failed business venture by her husband, she lost it all. Everything that they had worked for. With two children still at school, she became the family bread-winner. Eventually her marriage couldn't stand the strain and that crumbled also. There will be many women who will identify with her situation. The causes are not necessarily the same but the syndrome of the wife alone in mid-life after decades of marriage is increasingly common.

To say that Kendra fought back is an understatement. She not only got a full-time job, she also enrolled at university for a masters degree, graduating with distinction, she took up sailing and got her in-shore skippers certificate and she wrote two books. All this while battling ill health.

At fifty-four, there is little in Kendra's external demeanour to indicate the traumas of the past few years. She seems calm and relaxed and, now that she has found an even keel, revelling in her new life and achievements. But when she spoke of that terrible day, coinciding with the family's financial problems, when her balcony, holding over thirty women, collapsed twenty feet to the ground and there was not only the horror of crumpled and broken bodies but it also seemed symbolic of the fact that her whole life was collapsing around her, her voice broke with emotion and one was left in no doubt that the wounds are barely healed and the scars will last for a long time yet.

Kendra feels strongly that society is far too ready to consign older people to the scrapheap. Women in their fifties now are at the cutting edge. They are carving out careers, supporting families and taking on new interests. 'By and large, men get a bit more conservative as they age, while women get a real spurt on, especially sexually.'

Shortly after our meeting Kendra was due to visit China to advise that government on family planning issues, in particular, how informed choice might be substituted for Big Brother compulsion.

The invitation is an obvious tribute to her reputation and a challenge she relishes.

Kendra says that her mottos are that it is never too late for anything and life should be tackled on all cylinders. She is a living example of them both.

※ ※ ※

I was an only child, a much loved child, particularly by my father. I had a very close relationship with my father. My mother was a fairly flamboyant character. She was unpredictable, sort of a bohemian before the 1960s. She and her mother ran a very exclusive dress shop in Collins Street where they catered for the socialite women of the time. My mother spent any money that they made, I think, because she liked to live a very flamboyant life. I can remember stories of her going to the races in the country, the picnic races, in a taxi and having the taxi wait for her. In those days people didn't do those sort of things. I can remember when I was at school she would always turn up in some outrageous hat, much to my embarrassment.

I had a very happy childhood. I was a tomboy and I much preferred the company of boys. I loved school. I excelled at sport. I wasn't academic but I was always bright, I managed my school work very well, but boys were a bit of a distraction. It was only in the last year that I realised I needed to do something to pull myself together. I became a prefect and house captain and I took on the responsibility and started to work. I did very well in matriculation and won a scholarship to university which I deferred because I didn't really know what I wanted to do except I wanted to teach sport and my parents weren't very supportive about that.

I ended up doing nursing. Once I started nursing I just loved it, so I kept on. In a way, I suppose I missed an opportunity not going to university but I made up for it later in life.

My mother died very suddenly when I was nineteen. She became very ill with hepatitis and bronchial pneumonia. I was in Alice Springs on a holiday and I got a phone call to say that she had been taken to hospital and was dead on arrival. That was a huge crisis which I didn't deal with at the time, at all. I just blocked it out and got on with things. My father and I lived together, we were very close, and I just got on with my life. It wasn't until much later when I suffered a loss that it all came back and I had to deal with it then.

If I think about my life growing up as a young woman in suburban Melbourne it was very predictable. People had certain roles. I had a lot of freedom, my parents gave me a lot of freedom, and I spent a lot of time at the beach. I fell in love when I was thirteen. I had a very torrid romance from the age of thirteen to seventeen with the same person.

I pursued this person — he went to Melbourne Grammar — and we used to meet on the tram. It became a very physical relationship and very passionate. In those days, of course, I knew absolutely nothing about contraception. Nothing at all. It was the pre-pill days and in those days you didn't even see condoms, they were certainly not advertised. It was a very important relationship in my life and that distracted me from my schoolwork, I suppose, but he was gorgeous.

Thinking back about it now, we avoided penetration, but still I was always very conscious that there was a risk of getting pregnant, because my mother had had an abortion. Even though I wasn't supposed to know anything about it, and in those days it was illegal, I can remember my mother going to an abortionist in Toorak and having an abortion. I think probably because my father felt, or they both felt, that they couldn't afford it.

My parents didn't have a lot of money. My father was a commercial traveller with a cigarette company, and used to come home at the weekends. That caused a lot of strain for my mother because she was a party person. She loved going out so I think she had a few lovers. She was lonely, basically lonely. They separated briefly but they came back together again. My father was a very gentle man and had quite a lot to deal with, I think, with my mother. I felt guilty after my mother died that I hadn't been more understanding when she was ill. I didn't realise that she was ill and you are very selfish when you're young. I liked to think I was being myself and having a good time.

When I was growing up, I wanted my mother to be like everybody else's mother. I wanted her to be a sweet mother who didn't have mood swings, who wasn't a drama queen. She was flamboyant and that has had a big influence on me. I have always done things that have been a bit different. I have always been seen to do controversial things or be outspoken or different from my peers in some way.

I feel that for a long time I lived two lives. I was the perfect wife, the perfect mother, the well-bred, middle-class person with conservative values. But in my work I am not seen that way at all. I have often been called a radical feminist. Because I have worked in the area of sexuality and sex education I have always been outspoken about those things. I can remember at a dinner party in Melbourne talking about masturbation. The reason I was talking about it was because I had just had this amazing experience at work, at Family Planning. I was thrown into this area where I was dealing with people's sexuality and a woman who was on the board of Family Planning in Victoria came to speak at a course I was doing. She talked about the fact that one thing she did to help young men with cerebral palsy was to masturbate them to relieve their sexual tension and then she showed us a video on people masturbating. I remember sitting there, totally shocked. It was a new world for me. Although I had done nursing we never talked much about contraception or anything to do with sex. We used to sit in these lectures with stuffy old doctors who never talked to us about anything as basic as that. So it was a steep learning curve for me and I was so excited with all this new knowledge that I would talk about it with my friends who were shocked, because you didn't talk about those things in those days.

So because of my work I have become radical in one sense, but I have always been conservative in another, so I have had this feeling that there are two mes, until recently, when perhaps I am now more the radical me.

I went overseas when I finished nursing. Those were the days when you finished doing what you were doing and you went overseas for two years.

There was a group of us that lived together in London and some friends that I nursed with, who became really close friends and we have maintained that friendship for thirty-odd years. They are an amazing group of women. In all those years they have remained good friends, there has never been any bitchiness, they are there for each other. It has been a very strong group of women. I find it easy to be really intimate and close with women and I don't find it as easy to be that way with men. I have men friends but I can feel really close with my women friends, I can talk about anything and that is very important.

I met John the year after my mother died. Then I went overseas with a friend, on a Greek ship. What I didn't know when I was on that ship — I wondered why I felt so sick — I thought I was allergic to Greek food — but I was pregnant. When I got to Greece I had an abortion and that was very traumatic. At that time John had moved in with my father. Of course I didn't want my father to know and

John was begging me not to do it but I just couldn't have coped with a baby at that stage. It was pretty amazing having an abortion in a Greek hospital where nobody spoke my language. And it was traumatic because it was 1961.

John finally came over and it was hard but he convinced me that we should get married. We got married when I got back. I was twenty-three. Then we did all the things that people did. We saved up, bought a block of land and built a house. I worked for four years until we had saved up enough and we moved into the house the year that Mark, my son, was born and then another four years later I had Kate. I had a very conservative, very stable, middle-class Melbourne existence. Lovely, though, we had a lovely time. All our friends were marrying, and having children and we did the things that you did with your friends, like picnics and all that. It was great fun and then things became a bit tough because John was studying still. He was doing some extra qualifications and studying and then the job that he was in fell apart and he was out of work for six months. This is when the children were six and ten and he was out of work which was pretty hard because I wasn't working full-time then. He was offered a job in Sydney so we moved which was pretty traumatic because I had to leave behind my parents-in-law who I was very fond of, my father who had remarried, and my friends, and the house that we built, that we loved.

I knew I would have to work part-time because we wanted the children to go to private schools, which was going to cost money, and John couldn't afford it on his own. I either wanted to work in a hospital or family planning because I had been doing both in Melbourne. I always tried to do work where it didn't interfere with anybody else in the family, so at seven or eight o'clock at night I would take off and work a twelve-hour shift at the hospital, supervising two floors as a night sister, trying to keep my eyes open, checking drugs and things, and then drive home in the morning so that I would be there bright and fresh getting everybody off to school and doing the housework.

I was the classic *Women's Weekly* perfect mother and wife. My greatest compliment was when my friends would say, you could come to Kendra's house at nine o'clock in the morning and eat your meal off the kitchen floor. I had a spotless house, a spotless garden, won gardening competitions, everything was perfect. Perfect children, beautifully dressed. It was very important to me for everything to be just perfect and I had to do everything really well.

The other thing about being perfect in those days was you were very supportive of your husband, you were really important in his being a success. It was important for him to have a wife who was supportive, who relieved him of the stress when he came home from work. So I would tidy the house before he got home. He didn't like seeing any toys around the floor and you would try to have your children fed, so I would cook two meals every night. They would be all bathed and fed and the toys would be away and everything in the house would be absolutely pristine and he would come home and have to have a drink to let him unwind after his heavy day. Then I would cook a nice dinner.

My life has changed totally in the last nine years. My husband decided that he was going into his own business, much against my wishes, because when I was growing up we lived in a rented flat in Melbourne and one of the things I always wanted was to have a lovely house. We had that in Melbourne, we worked really hard and built a lovely house. Then when we came to Sydney we bought a really nice house and I took great pride in it, furnishing it and painting it and gardening. I did everything around the house including repairing the roof, guttering, concreting, everything. My home was really important to me. Then John decided he would go into business with a man whom I instinctively didn't trust. I think men can be really naive and because this fellow worked for John he thought it would be fine. But I was very apprehensive about it right from the start and I begged him not to do it because I felt we had too much to lose. I can remember sitting around the kitchen table with John talking about the finances. Because of the roles we had he had always handled the money side. Any money I earned I had just bought the children clothes and the luxuries and I had let him handle everything, I suppose because I thought I couldn't do it very well. But I knew this was wrong. And it turned out to be a total disaster because within a year the fellow pulled out. John had put all our money in, everything, and on Christmas Eve, the fellow left John a note saying he was pulling out and of course he hadn't put his money in. From that moment on our life just took a turn. I had two children at private schools, so I went to work full-time. In the past my work had always been just something extra, but then I became the breadwinner for the family.

It was extremely tough and of course our relationship suffered because John is a very proud person. We just couldn't talk. We knew what was happening and I knew we were going to lose the house, I knew we were going to lose absolutely everything, literally everything that we had worked for all those years, and it was pretty tough.

At that time I had suffered a series of losses as well. It is funny how symbolic things happen. About a year earlier I was the class mother for my son's class at school. I had a morning tea for about eighty women from the school plus the headmaster's wife. It was a beautiful day and I had all these women on the deck out among the trees. All of a sudden, one minute there were thirty-five women on the deck and the next minute there were none. The whole deck collapsed. My house suddenly became a battlefield. We had women bleeding and towels and women fainting. There were three or four nurses there who went into automatic pilot and I apparently rang the ambulance although I don't remember it at all. The headmaster's wife was just about to give a speech and all of a sudden, they disappeared. The deck just went *choong*. It was about twenty feet from the ground. In a way it was symbolic. I don't like metaphors and symbols, but it was symbolic because from that moment on my life was totally different. Everything started to fall apart.

When I went to work full-time is when I started to get a bit of confidence in myself, because I had lived vicariously through my husband and my children. Their successes were my successes, when they did something it was great for me and also their failures were my failures. I felt that my work was peripheral to my life because, although I enjoyed it, it was not central to what I was there for. But from when I started to work full-time, I began to carve out a bit of a niche for myself. I realised that I had a lot of energy and creativity that I hadn't known about until I was out there and had to do it. A lot of dramatic things happened to me after that.

This was in 1985–86 and because of my work in family planning and sexual health, I was offered a position in a newly formed consultancy looking at ways of educating youth about the dangers of AIDS. As a result of that I ended up working in the Health Department full-time as an AIDS education officer. There was a lot of hysteria around at the time and it was a very stressful job for me. I was there for about eighteen months and my job was to run training programs for doctors and nurses and health professionals in rural areas, so I had to go to the country quite a lot. There was so much hysteria and I had to educate my department, ambulance officers, all the services and, at the same time as I was doing this very stressful job, my life was falling apart. I was working full-time, my husband was trying to keep his business going by himself, so he was never there, and I had children at school. It was a nightmare. At the same time I became very ill, and in the middle of all of this my father died in Melbourne from a stroke. He lived about six weeks so I was back and forth to Melbourne. I was bleeding heavily all the time for about two years because I had fibroids but I really didn't have time to be sick. Each month I would just about bleed to death and of course as a result of that I got really ill. Then I found I had to have a hysterectomy. So in the space of about two years I lost my father, I had a hysterectomy, I knew we were going to lose the house, and my relationship was absolutely nowhere. I was forty-seven then and my mother had died when she was forty-seven. My daughter went to Alice Springs on a holiday and

I had been in Alice Springs when I learned that my mother died. With the combination of all those things, I went down like a ton of bricks. I was really depressed. I eventually got some help, counselling help. That helped me a lot to get some belief in my own strength, my own ability.

I knew that I was going to have to keep going and I am a person that if things are bad I have to do something, I am a doer. I thought, okay, I am going to have to support myself and probably a family for the rest of my life. I have been teaching for eighteen years and I don't actually have any formal qualifications. So I enrolled at Sydney University to do a graduate diploma, followed by a masters degree in Health Science Education. I was working full-time as well and I graduated in 1992 with distinction. I absolutely sailed through that course. One year I did eight subjects and I got distinctions all the way through. That was satisfying for me because I had put university on hold when I was young.

As part of my course I had to make a video. I had never made a video, I didn't even know how to hold a camera. But I made a promotional video for Family Planning where I did everything. I was the camera person, I did the editing, I was the voice-over person, I did everything. All of a sudden I thought, I can do anything. I found that people were wanting me to speak at conferences and then I was approached by a publisher to write a book about menopause, part of a health book series. I can remember going to this book publisher and thinking, what am I doing here? But they seemed to think that I could do it and I thought, well, if they think I can do it, okay, I can do it. And I did. This was on top of my study for my masters and working full-time. I used to write at night — start about nine o'clock and write through for three or four hours. So, it's a small book.

Then I wrote another book on contraception. The menopause book is in its third reprint. It's doing really well, selling all over the world. It's only a small $10 health book but it's part of a health book series and I did that.

John tried everything he possibly could to keep going but I knew that we were going to lose everything. Being a man, he couldn't talk about it because he felt so devastated and we got to the stage where we couldn't talk about it either. We had to have a mortgagee's auction. That was terrible, we had people coming and saying they were going to take all the furniture, and the nightmare of trying to keep going. We did lose the house, we did lose absolutely everything and up until a week before we had to move out of the house John and I hadn't actually sat down and talked about whether we were going to stay together or whether we weren't. It was just unbelievable: a couple who had lived together, been together, for thirty years. He was part of my life and I was part of his, but we were like children, we couldn't talk about it. It was terrible. In the end he said, 'I can't face the blame, I can't live with the blame.' Then I had to think, what am I going to do? A friend took me around looking at flats and that was depressing too, because having grown up in a flat I thought, I just can't cope with it. John helped me move and he and I kissed each other goodbye and we both cried, he broke down and I broke down, and that was the end of our relationship. We're still friends, I see him quite frequently but we are still unable to talk about what happened.

We're not divorced. It's on hold. It's funny, it's just that he has been such a part of my life. I don't think we could ever live together again because I seem to have moved on. It was like a liberation in a way. It was traumatic but I got this tremendous creative surge. All of a sudden there is this turning point where you have given everything, your all, to everybody else and then, there you are, you can do what you want to do. I did so much in those few years. I got my masters degree and I wrote two books and I spoke all over Australia. I am a good speaker and I can motivate people in terms of women's health. I am often asked to go to the country, to do consultancies, for various health projects and things. I have just been approached by the World Health Organisation and I am going to China in September to run a training course for doctors and nurses who don't speak English, on communication counselling and family planning, which is a huge challenge because China has their one-child policy. They're used to telling people what to do. I have been asked to try and shift them from telling to facilitating people's choices about contraception. That is an enormous challenge. I am continually amazed at how people keep asking me to do things. In the last few years doors just keep opening.

The other thing I did, I wanted to learn to sail, so I enrolled at the Australian Sailing School. I did the beginners' course and then I enrolled in the competent crews' course and I sat my theory exam and I have got my in-shore skippers certificate. I don't think I would have done those things if I was as I imagined I would be at my age. I had this vision — you get married and you have children and you live happily ever after. I am just having a totally different life.

I think sex roles are changing, which is good, but I think women will always do more, because of their nurturing, caring side. I wanted to bring my son up with the values that I had, but I can see, even with my children, that I let my son get away with far more than I let my daughter get away with. I beat myself up about that a bit. My son lives in a house in Balmain with some friends. He relates very well to women, he is very good with women, but I think I could have done a better job with him, I could have worked on him a bit harder. I let him get away with a bit too much. I am hoping that he won't take on some of the attitudes he saw in the house, but that might be a bit of a wish.

I think my daughter will definitely be more demanding in her relationships because she has seen some of the things that I have fought against and so she will expect more. She will be a lot tougher than I was.

A lot of older women find it hard to think of themselves as being sexually attractive any more and that can be a bit daunting, particularly for women in new relationships. I can identify with that. I was in a relationship for thirty years and now I am on my own. I would feel pretty vulnerable, and I have talked to other women too, about exposing your body for the first time to a new partner and you know your body isn't as great as it was. One of the things that happens to women as they get older is that they do put on weight. It's harder to lose weight and your body shape changes. The fat gets redistributed around your body. And, as you walk down the street, men don't look at you as much as maybe they once would. You hear an odd wolf whistle occasionally and you look around to find, well, it's not me. So I think some women don't feel as sexual as they were. You also see that a lot of older men, to restore their belief in their own virility or enhance their sexual performance, take up with younger women. I think the chances of older women having relationships with younger men are not as likely, although this might be changing slightly. I remember seeing, last year, a *Women's Weekly* cover of Maggie Tabberer with her lover and I thought, oh, that's a lovely photo, and I looked at the headline and it said, OLDER WOMAN, YOUNGER MAN — HOW DOES SHE COPE? I thought that was outrageous, it should have been HOW DOES HE COPE?, because she is so vital. That's the way society looks at older women. The other thing is older women on television. There aren't the role models and the ones that are there, they are often the Joan Collins types, the ones who work on their looks every minute of the day. They don't pay the money for women television presenters if they've got grey hair. They just gradually go off the television once they are not perceived as being sexually desirable and they are showing their age, whereas men can be there with their hair transplants and they go on forever.

Among my women friends, one woman I know is divorced and has always been very successful with men. Even now, she is able to attract men and I asked her how she did it, what her secret was. She said, 'It's easy, you just sit there and ask them about themselves and every time they say something, you say, "Oh, you're wonderful, you're so clever."' I thought, I can't be bothered with that. Men probably get a bit intimidated with me. I am actually interested in men's things, I love talking about business but, I suppose, in a way I have forgotten what it is like to flirt with men and I don't think I could be bothered. So if I ever do meet somebody it will have to be somebody pretty special. I just don't think I could be bothered playing all those games any more.

There are occasions when I watch a video or a romantic film or movie and I think, wouldn't it be nice to walk along the beach and to have a male companion to talk to. I miss that intimacy, I suppose. But I've seen women who are in relationships who don't have it anyway. They're in a committed relationship but they are actually as if they are on their own. I have been in that situation myself, where there isn't that communication. One of the benefits I have now is freedom to do exactly what I want to do and I have never had that before. I am really enjoying it. But I don't know if I want to do that for ever. Maybe I will find somebody to spend the rest of my life with and maybe I won't, but I am not looking.

For women who have placed a lot of importance on their body and their looks the visible signs of ageing can be quite devastating. You see that with women having face-lifts and tummy tucks and putting themselves under the knife. I am really interested in hormone replacement therapy and the fact that they market it to women by looking at what women worry about most. They talk about it improving your skin and your hair and your sexual performance and things like that, and a lot of women clutch on to it in the hope that it is somehow going to keep them youthful. It does have health benefits for some women, but it's not something that all women need, although that's the way the drug companies would like to see it because it's a huge market. The fastest growing age group in the world is women in their eighties. Older women are a big potential marketing group so you'll find a lot of products and things being marketed towards older women.

Physical frailty is one of the things that does frighten me. Last year I got quite ill. I got hepatitis, which is interesting because my mother died of hepatitis, and I was very ill for six weeks. I was flat on my back for six weeks, couldn't move, and I felt really frightened because I couldn't work. I kept thinking, I have no financial security any more, I have lost everything, I have my work and if I can't work what will I do? That was pretty frightening. But when I am busy and active I feel I can do anything and that's how I feel at the moment. I don't smoke any more, I exercise, I watch what I eat, I don't drink very much and I feel healthier now than I have ever felt.

Men or women can be sexually active and continue to have a sexual relationship until the moment they die. Sexuality changes, sensuality becomes more important than the actual physical sexual intercourse act. Especially for people in a close relationship, as they get older the need for touching is really important. That is one of the things I miss most of all — touching — so I go and have a massage once a month. Somebody asked me recently what I miss most about not being in a relationship. I miss the body in the bed and I miss the touching. So I think that sexuality changes as people get older. Their need to be touched and the sensuality is really important but the physical performance side of it is not so important. And there are physical changes through illness or drugs that people are on as they get older. A lot of heart drugs and other drugs have side effects on sexual performance. A lot of those things aren't talked about much and people get a bit frightened.

There is a lot of pressure on men as they get older. In terms of being a man you've got to be able to perform and obviously older men can't. Although the minute the man can't perform, the woman says, well it must be me, that extra roll of flab around my stomach, I'm not really turning him on. We always think it is our fault. But really it is something that is just a process of getting older and the focus needs to be a bit different.

I think women become more sexually assertive as they get older. They are able to get their needs met, while perhaps in the past they haven't been able to and that puts pressure on men too. Men have grown up thinking they're the ones who are in control, they're the ones who know instinctively what to do, and if they get told they are not doing it properly then they feel that they are inadequate as a lover, so they feel a bit threatened by older women who tell them to lift their game.

I think getting older is harder for men than for women. I see men that I've known for many years and I think it's very hard for men, particularly men who haven't got to the top of their career. A lot of men have been losing their jobs or businesses or whatever and they don't feel good about themselves as men. Women are more resourceful. When you're a mother and wife and you've got to do fifty million things at once and you are used to thinking laterally, you are not focused on just one thing. Consequently when situations change, women can adapt more quickly and think of different things to do, whereas men often can only think of the thing that they have always done. It is hard for men to have a career change or to totally change. Some men can do it but it doesn't come as easily to them and they can't admit to other men that they have been a failure.

A lot of men get softer and the feminine side of their nature can be expressed more as they get older. It's interesting because I find women become more assertive and yet men get a bit softer. They say that as we age we get more like each other and perhaps we do. I think women's testosterone levels run riot too — of course, we've got testosterone as well as oestrogen — and the testosterone gives you this assertiveness and drive and sexual energy.

For me the most striking thing about being in my fifties is freedom. Freedom to do exactly what I want to do. I just feel free and I don't have to worry so much about everybody else. I can enjoy things. I am finding I am enjoying the energy and the creativity. I have this pool of energy and creativity that I suppose had been submerged for many years and I feel I can let it all out now. I feel more confident. I feel extremely confident of my abilities. I feel I can do anything, absolutely anything. Nothing fazes me, I am not frightened any more of anything. I feel a strength within myself that I didn't feel before when I felt I needed to be protected by a man or I had to have somebody there who was stronger than I was to make decisions. I can remember when I had to lease a car for myself. I had never done anything like that before but once I had done it, I knew I could do it. Then I had to go and talk to the bank manager. I had never done that before and once you've done it you can do it, it's not a big deal. But when you've always had somebody making those decisions for you, handling those things for you, you feel that you can't do them. I know now I can, I can do anything really.

I don't feel I'm ready to be old at all. I feel very energetic. I have much more energy than I can ever remember having.

I do feel that if I had started it all ten years earlier it would have been better. I feel that I have to do everything very quickly because I didn't have that opportunity before. Time is running out. But then maybe I needed to have these experiences, perhaps I needed to go through this to enable me to get here, to where I am now. Maturity is one thing. I don't think I have actually grown up yet. There's a child in me still, I think. I don't think I'm really grown up yet, but I am getting there.

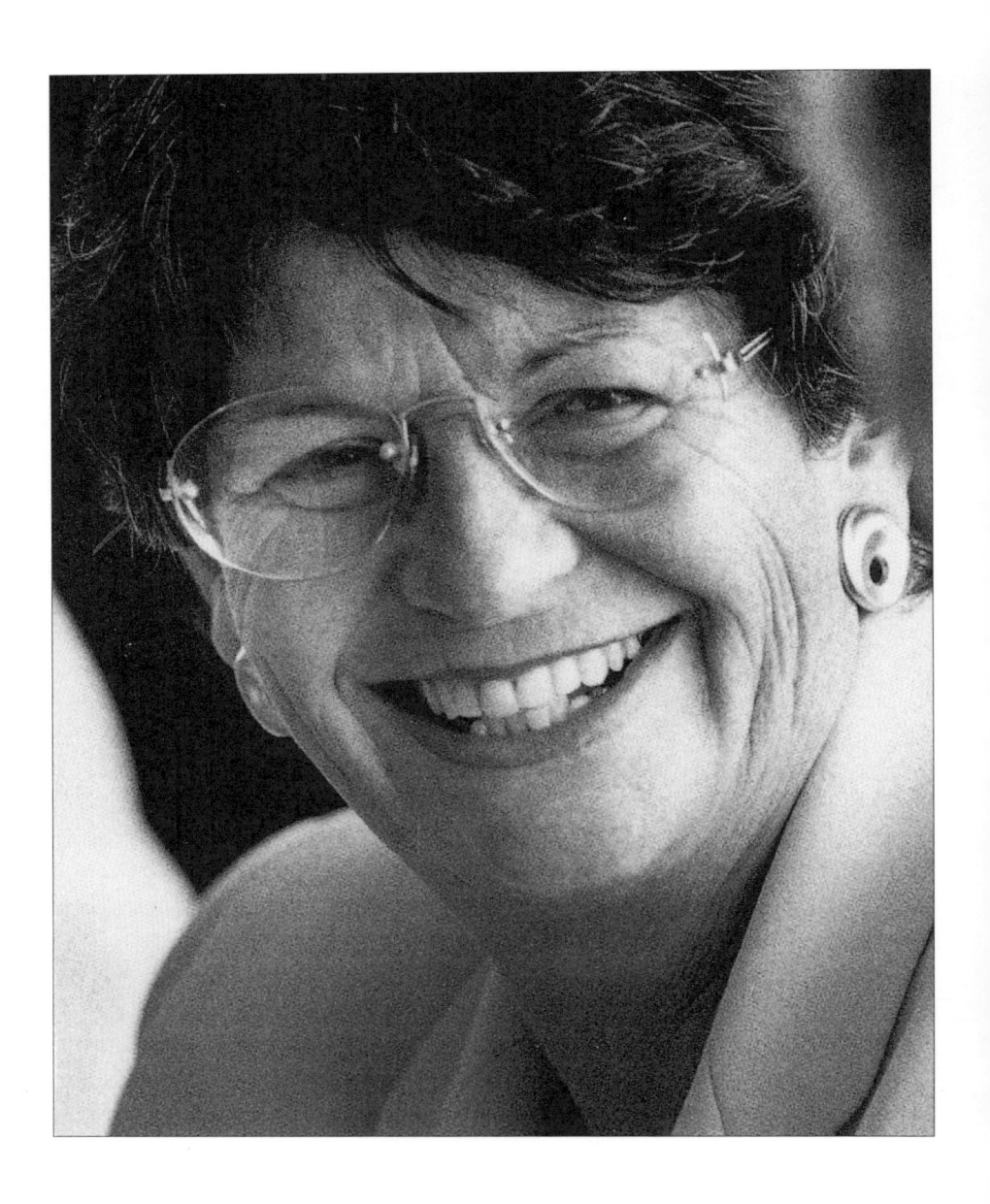

*I can't remember ever having enjoyed myself so much as I am right now.
There's such a balance and everything I'm doing I am enjoying. There are no 'shoulds'
there at all.*

❖ ❖ ❖

Eve Mahlab

It was hard not to feel envious of a woman like Eve who really has managed to have her cake and eat it too. A successful business of her own, a happy marriage, a good relationship with her independent kids and a commitment to other women and their struggle.

Tall Poppies, Susan Mitchell, Penguin Books, 1984

Eve Mahlab is a dear and valued friend of many years. When I asked if she would agree to be included in the book, there was no doubt in my mind that her approach to the topic would be different, and I was not disappointed. Eve's primary concern was not to say how good the fifties are for her, though she acknowledged that to be the case, but was, as it has always been, to look at the situation from the point of view of all women, the 'non-winners' as well as the 'winners', and make the point that for many women turning fifty is not something to be celebrated. For women who have inadequate financial resources or whose health is poor or who are alone, the fact of being no longer young is a time of extreme difficulty and a precursor of an old age they cannot do other than dread.

Eve's life story has already been well documented. As readers of *Tall Poppies* will know, she came to Melbourne as a small child with her Jewish parents fleeing Nazi Europe. After a childhood in which she says she was always conscious of being different, she did law at the insistence of her father who, she wryly recalls, had the view that she was very difficult, very outspoken, very independent and would never find a man to put up with her. She would therefore have to support herself.

At twenty-one, after a postgraduation overseas trip, she escaped family pressures by running away to Sydney where she met her husband, Frank. She says that they decided to marry a week after they met. After having three children in three and a half years, Eve decided that unrelieved domesticity was not for her and sought part-time work as a lawyer. The difficulties that entailed led her to establish an agency specialising in the placement of other married women lawyers who wanted to combine the raising of a family with outside work, and so began a very successful business career. As time went on she diversified and expanded, building a substantial national business in human resources and publishing, with a particular emphasis on business diaries. In 1982 Eve was named Businesswoman of the Year and in 1988 she was made an Officer of the Order of Australia for services to business, government and the community, particularly women.

In the 1970s Eve joined the Women's Electoral Lobby and became one of the the most prominent feminists in the country. Blindingly intelligent and highly articulate, she was often called on to talk to the media and to groups and in general to be the public face of the movement for women's rights.

Twenty years later, Eve is not quite so much in the limelight. She says that she has lost some of her anger although, if that is so, after half an hour's conversation it is difficult to believe that she has lost much of it. She points out that women are still discriminated against, still among the poorest groups in society, and she seems just as passionately committed as she ever was to redressing the balance.

One area where she has changed is in her attitude to matters domestic. When I rang to make an appointment to see her, her office referred me to her daughter's home. A flustered-sounding Eve answered the phone and said, 'I'll have to ring you back, I've left the side of the cot down!' Minding her grandson! In the middle of the working week! This was not the Eve Mahlab I had known.

Fundamentally an entrepreneur and always looking for new challenges, a few years ago Eve executive-produced a television documentary, Not a Bedroom War, dealing with women and leadership, based on an international conference held in Ireland. It was shown on SBS television and short-listed for the United Nations Media Peace Prize. She describes it as one of the most satisfying things she has ever done. I recall at the time saying that I had not known she had the skills to be a TV producer. She said she hadn't, it was just something she wanted to do, thought was worth doing, and so she set about finding a way to do it.

Still in the vanguard of achievement, about two years ago Eve became one of a handful of women in Australia to join the board of a major company with her appointment as a director of Westpac. She also currently serves on the Victorian State Training (TAFE) board, the Walter and Eliza Hall Institute of Medical Research, the Jewish Commission for the Future and Open Channel.

Eve does seem to have it all. Still in an obviously happy marriage after thirty-five or so years, stepping back now from intense business involvement to pursue other, broader interests, close to her adult children and relishing her role as grandmother, perhaps she is a target for envy. But she has worked for what she has. It hasn't all just happened and nor has it all been smooth sailing.

Apart from an extraordinary generosity of spirit, the quality in Eve that I have always admired and found intriguing is her ability to analyse exactly what it is she wants and then to focus on getting there. There is a clarity about her thought processes and a strength of purpose which is rare. Many of us just find it easier to make excuses, to bow out if it is too hard. I have never heard Eve Mahlab make an excuse, she simply gets in there and does it. If she can't do it she moves in a different direction and doesn't waste time and energy on the impossible. Envy has a certain 'if only' quality: 'If only things had been different, I could have had all that.' Eve has had as many hurdles to overcome as most of us. She deserves her success.

✥ ✥ ✥

I think it is important to say that the fifties are not fabulous for many, many women. In fact, it might be that the fifties aren't fabulous for most women. They're fabulous for me, so far, because I'm financially secure, I'm healthy and I'm loved. I think that all those things are absolutely essential and it remains an undebatable fact that not all women enjoy good health, many women are alone, and many, many women in their fifties are not financially secure.

I have just been on a women business leaders' mission in Singapore which had about a hundred of the most successful women from Australia in conference with a hundred of the most successful women leaders in business from the ASEAN countries. Apart from a few, almost token words acknowledging that development has to be equally enjoyed by men and women, there was virtually no recognition that women are still the most disadvantaged people in societies all over the world. Women still make up the majority of the poor and the majority of refugees. The conference was all about success and how women are the factors of production and have to be respected and all that sort of thing and it didn't measure and didn't relate at all to the women at the bottom. It was about women at the top.

I think that there is an unfortunate trend in moving away from thinking of women as victims. With the women's movement in the 1970s what we did was point out the many inequities and problems that women had in society. Now there seems to me to be a reaction to that and women only want to be portrayed as winners. That's all very well, because a victim mentality is undermining. But the truth is that very many women *are* victims and society does not treat them equally. This inequality begins to be felt even more as women age. Whilst I am particularly fortunate, I have amongst my friends many women who don't think the fifties are fabulous at all. These are women who are not healthy. Also, the statistics show that only ten per cent of women earn more than $32 000 a year. This indicates that by the time women are fifty, unless they have a partner and together they have shared the costs of raising children, they have very little in savings or in assets. If women have been single parents, either as a result of divorce or widowhood, and have brought up children on their own, this has depleted their resources.

I also think there is something more subtle going on which has analogies with the early 1970s. Many of the prominent women are seen as successful women, and they are assumed not to have any financial problems. They are busy filling the role of superwoman and I suspect that they have financial problems looming up ahead of them which are fearful, but they are not speaking out about it. I think there is a need for some sort of group to lobby for changes or to prevent changes which might disadvantage them further than they are already disadvantaged. For instance, many of these women were excluded from superannuation schemes in the companies that they worked for for much of their life because it is only recently that superannuation was removed from the exclusion part of the Sex Discrimination Act. Also, for some of these women their pattern of employment was different because they moved from job to job. Apart from that, most women have been employed in small businesses where they don't have superannuation and the business doesn't pay much in any other way. So you've got this whole body of women who are now assumed to be terribly well off who really are not well off at all.

I certainly think there is a need for activism on behalf of older women. Whilst there are groups of various kinds, I am not sure that they are politically assertive or politically astute. I think there should be much more activism on a sophisticated political level as there was for women generally in the early 1970s. I don't see that happening to any great extent. The postponement of the age of eligibility for the pension so that it is the same as for men is an example of the failure of political action. It is totally inequitable for women to be treated the same as men when they haven't had an equal opportunity to earn the same. Plus, women get squeezed out of the workforce much earlier than men, in their early fifties when they are no longer young and beautiful. To make them eke out a living and live on any savings they have until they get the pension at sixty-five is an outrage.

Women are the only group that get more radical as they get older. Many young women of ability, particularly those working in the private sector, feel there is no need for political activism. It is quite easy if you have been privileged and have a good education to feel today, when you are young, that you can have it all. Young women have not suffered, they don't really know what it's like as you get older with all the disadvantages and all the problems that come when you get married, when you have children, and still want to earn an income. It is only as you get older that you realise you haven't got all the answers and therefore we should be very, very careful. Women like me can keep talking, keep reminding them that we are talented and we are privileged and that's just not life for most people. We should always listen to the young, but older women should not abdicate or accept that life is always fabulous.

I don't know enough about what the Women's Electoral Lobby is doing right now but it is my general experience that organisations tend to get slightly stale. They are fuelled by the passions of the people who set them up. It may be that the Women's Electoral Lobby does have a sub-committee which is passionate about this issue but, as far as I know, that does not exist. It would be very good if a group of women who felt passionate about this issue did band together and did start doing the research and lobbying necessary but, above all, gave a voice to this particular group of women. It should be easier now because most women are much more sophisticated about the law and political lobbying.

I myself am not politically active any more. I do a lot of public speaking which is fuelled by my feminism and I see myself as a catalyst for other women but I am just not there in the front line now. I don't particularly want to be in the front line.

I think that as I have got older I have got more selfish. I also think that I have lost some of the energy I had in those early years. Some of my anger has gone, although I can still get angry. I remained a member but I stopped being active in the Women's Electoral Lobby in the early 1980s. I tried to go back a couple of times but it just didn't work for me and there hasn't been another organisation that has excited me in the way that WEL did. I have recently got involved with the Key Centre for Women's Health at Melbourne University and have established a strategy committee to market the centre and ultimately raise funds for it. The centre is unique in that it blends medicine with social research and, above all, it listens to women about their experiences. That excites me, but it is not political.

It is possible that some people don't want to be connected with groups identified with older women because it is likely to rebound on them, for example, in their jobs. I think it's not realistic to feel that way. It reminds me a bit of the women in the early 1970s who said, I don't want to be a woman, I just want to be a person, but the fact was that all the society out there regarded them as a woman. If you are an older woman, and if you are ageing, that's how society sees you, irrespective of whether you draw attention to it or not.

Anyway, I don't see that it is much better to be seen as forty-plus than fifty-plus. If you are a woman and you are over that nubile twenty-plus or maybe early thirties there is a perception that you are old anyway and you become marginalised. Individual women can work against that marginalisation with more or less success — by the time you are fifty, alright, you can work on it so that people only think you are forty — but I don't think that helps much at all. It is much better, as we did in the early 1970s, coming out and saying, yeah, I'm an old woman, and old women have something to contribute, and I want to be proud of being an old woman, and look at me, take me seriously.

One of the most important political issues for older women is superannuation where we have been treated very, very badly. Apart from the aspects I mentioned before in relation to successful women who I suspect have unrecognised problems, I think women in general have been sold a bill of goods in that superannuation is not a solution for low-income people and most women are low-income earners. Basically, low-income earners have been deprived of wages that they need, in the present, and been forced to save, when they can't afford to save, for pay-outs some time in the future. Most of the money goes in administration costs to other people anyway. I think low-income people are entitled to have all their income as they earn it and still get pensions when they are older. Superannuation is regressive and it benefits high-income earners and men in particular.

All the sorts of economic rationalist things that make things difficult for low-income people affect women disproportionately. Most of the poor are older women. My generation in particular is very badly off because most of the women of my age group were still brought up to believe that they would be looked after by men. At least the coming generations have got skills and the expectation of working and earning their own living, but at my age many of the women haven't got those skills and are financially in a very insecure position.

Moving away from the financial side, although it still has a financial element, I know many women in their fifties who are caring for elderly parents who are in their eighties and it seems that for them they will spend more of their life looking after dependent parents than they ever spent looking after dependent children. That is the reality too for many women in their fifties.

Then as you get older you get invisible and so you are not only not seen but your problems are not heard. Older women are the most overlooked and invisible group in our society. And there are so many jokes. Even the stereotype, 'an old woman', is such a putdown. Whilst it may be improving as older women assert themselves, basically, most attitudes to older women are negative.

The other thing that I have noticed among some of my friends in their fifties is that they really do miss having sex in their lives. The ones who are single find that they are no longer attractive to men, they find it really hard to find casual or permanent partners and they just miss it. From a social point of view many of these women find that they are not lonely, in fact, they get tremendous social interaction from other women, but several have told me that they miss sex. I thought that perhaps you could have brothels for women but when I suggest it no one actually jumps for joy at the prospect. Until men stop being attracted only to women who are younger or less powerful than they are and they see the beauty of older women, I don't see any way out of it.

There are good things about getting older though, which depend very much on those factors that I mentioned earlier — a certain degree of financial security, good health, good relationships and meaningful activity. When you get to fifty you don't care so much about what people think, you wear the clothes that you are comfortable in, rather than thinking about how you look, and you accept yourself for who you are. You know it's highly unlikely that if you diet, if you read, if you use this shampoo or that, that you're really going to improve yourself all that much and it really doesn't matter any more whether you do. You know you are being taken for who you are for better or worse and that's it. On my fiftieth birthday I stopped wearing high heels. It's very liberating!

I sold my business in 1987 because I felt, rightly or wrongly, that I could not myself build that business any more. It required skills other than the ones I had. I would have had to move into professional management and I always liked the close contact with the people I worked with. I felt that if I couldn't build it I didn't want to stay in it. Also, it was a time when businesses were being sold for extraordinary amounts and I knew I would never get another offer like that. I had no ambivalence about it. I discussed it with Frank and we believed it would free me up to do other things. I didn't know quite what they would be, but I just thought it was time to move on.

Since then I've executive-produced a film on women and leadership called *Not a Bedroom War* which has given me an enormous amount of pleasure. The producers were Anne Deveson and Anna Grieve and it was directed by Kay Pavlov. I just feel like bursting with pride every time I see it. It was shown on SBS a couple of times. I have had more time for boards so there have been community boards, and of course there's Westpac. Westpac has been an absolutely huge growth experience for me which I just love. I have a lot more spare time and that's been absolutely beaut. I have renewed relationships with friends and family that I just didn't have time for before. Most of all I have time to think and I like staring into space and thinking. I like just thinking about issues and having time to think before I open my mouth. Frank says it's because I like playing God.

Feminism and power are the two things that are on my mind. Usually the things I think about are prompted by being asked to speak on some topic and then I start 'nudging' around it. People are now fascinated about what it's like to be on a corporate board like Westpac. What do they do on boards? How do people get to be on boards? Lots and lots of women have rung me up and said that they would like board appointments and could I advise them as to how to do it. So I start thinking about what is the path towards board appointments and 'why me?' because I am not a conventional board appointment. I haven't lived the corporate life and I haven't been a chief executive in a major company or any of those things. Why was I invited? I think basically because I am an independent, lateral thinker and intelligent and outspoken and because some corporations are wanting to change their culture to optimise the skills of women. In the post-industrial age, brains become much more important than brawn and women have fifty per cent of the brain power so we are an under-utilised resource. A few women have been there in the large corporations showing what we can do, so more advanced companies are starting to understand how much more can be achieved if only they can find and attract good women. I think because I have always been very articulate in this area, I've become a sort of symbol of what the company wants to do.

I think my main contribution is that I am an outsider and I don't travel on the same assumptions as men. I ask questions that they don't ask. I ask questions about things that they take for granted and sometimes the questions need to be asked – although of course sometimes they don't and then you feel like an idiot, but that's the chance you take. Another thing I do is informalise the proceedings. I don't know whether it's me or the fact that I'm a woman but I think it leads to more discussion, more bouncing off each other, makes it more relaxed. Also, I approach things in different ways because of my small business background. I'm very attuned to practical, hands-on factors. As a woman, I'm less intimidating, and I try to build communication bridges.

The present chief executive of Westpac puts a value on cultural diversity. He comes from an American bank where sixty per cent of the managers were women and Westpac had three per cent or something like that. He can see the value that women add. So Westpac is a very exciting place to be right now. It's very satisfying for me because I can see all the human resources things that I have ever talked about being put into practice. I think it's a great fit. I'm good for them and they're good for me. And I like them. I always had this feeling of not being absolutely comfortable with the corporate scene and there are lots of companies whose business activities are actually harmful or at least just not worthwhile doing. But banking, in a capitalist society, which is channelling capital from people who have it to people who don't so they can build their personal wealth by buying homes or building businesses, is a really good thing to be doing. So you start with doing something worthwhile and try to do it in a profitable and ethical way.

I'm having a fantastic time. For me the fifties really are fabulous. I can't remember ever having enjoyed myself so much as I am right now. There's such a balance and everything I'm doing I am enjoying. There are no 'shoulds' there at all. Every now and then I get so scared because I'm afraid it will end or I won't have enough time to enjoy it for long. You get greedy. You want it to go on for ever.

Most of the time, I don't worry about getting older. I don't even worry much about getting frail. I have a wonderful role model in my mother who is extraordinary. She's eighty-three and she still goes overseas by herself every year. She plays golf a couple of days a week. She is getting frailer and this year she ordered a wheelchair at the various airports — because she doesn't just go to one place — and she said, 'Do you think they'll mind, giving me a wheelchair when they see I've brought my golf clubs?'! She's absolutely terrific.

On the other hand, she has always fretted about 'looking' old. She is very realistic and she says that society doesn't value old women. It is important for older women to work on raising the status of 'old' rather than trying to look young. I love the badge that older feminists in the US wear that says, HOW DARE YOU THINK I'D RATHER LOOK YOUNG? And I love Gloria Steinem's reply to someone who told her she didn't look fifty-seven and she said, 'This is what fifty-seven looks like.'

With my kids, like all parents there have been very rough times along the way. But I feel now that they are moving into their thirties the relationships are good with all of them. I feel good about that, that we have been able to maintain those relationships. Frank and I are comfortable and enjoy each other. They say that life begins when the kids leave home and the dog dies!

My daughter Karen bought a small part of my business. I get enormous pleasure that the business is going into the second generation and that she and her husband can build it beyond where I could ever build it. I like that concept of growth and continuity.

I love my grandchild absolutely. Having children was a really serious business. I was very conscious that I hadn't got as much out of the childhood of my children as I could have. At the time I undervalued the joys of parenting. It was a serious responsibility to bring up children and I wasn't relaxed about it in the way my daughter is. I started enjoying it when I went back to work and I wasn't so insecure any more. So I was absolutely determined to enjoy my grandchild and I have him every Tuesday afternoon. We do things together and just watching him and thinking about how he learns to walk and talk and how he tries to communicate and what sort of person he is — it's absolutely fascinating. When he sees me and opens his arms — it's just wonderful.

I think of myself as successful, but I've never measured it in terms of public success the way men do. I think it's always been a side product of doing something that you really want to do and care about. I have enough money to live on, work that is meaningful and someone to share my life with. That's success.

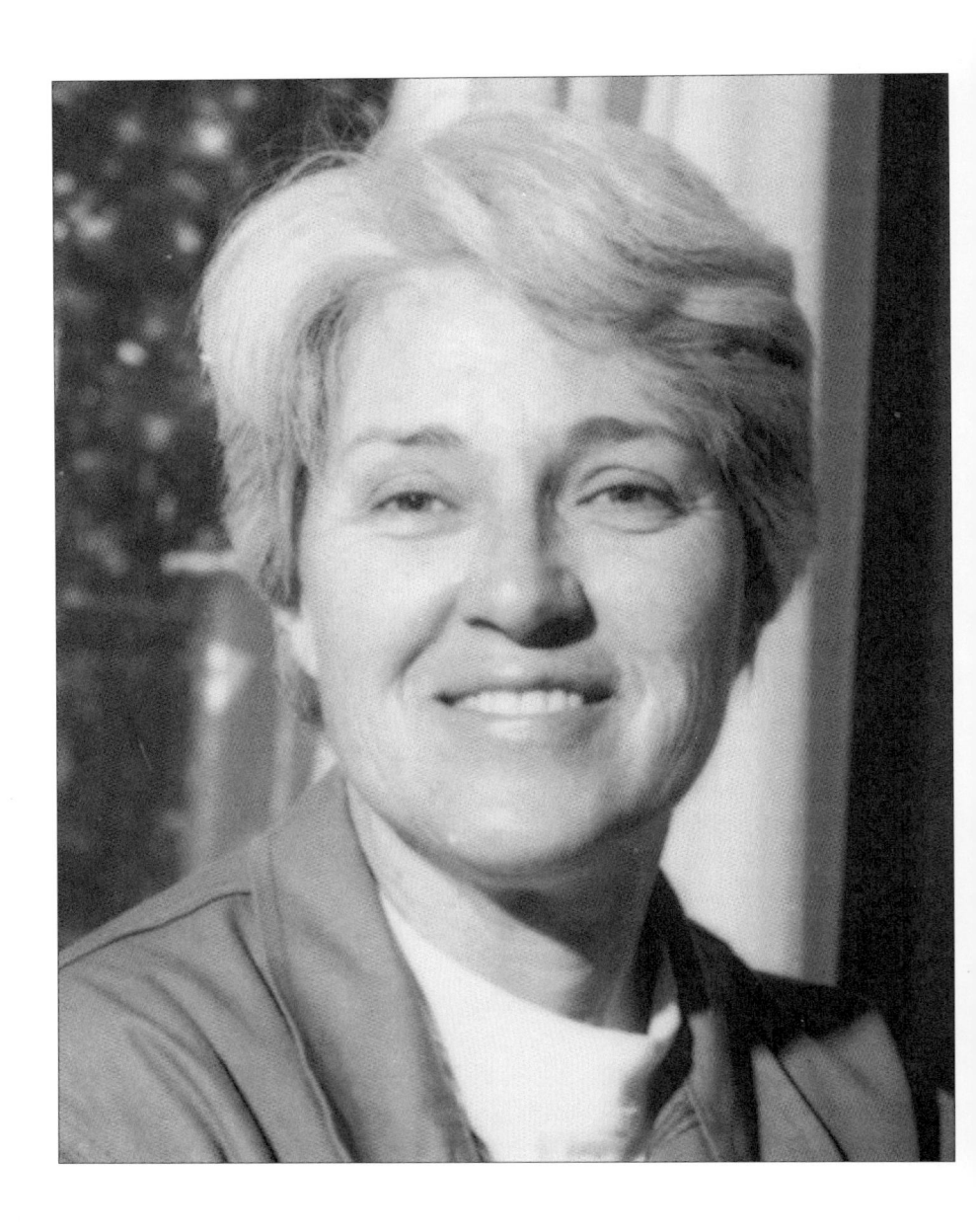

I think the most striking thing about being in your fifties is being able to see the past and the future. There is a moment when you stop. It is almost as though you are given the time to stop and see where you have come from, what the future possibly holds.

❖ ❖ ❖

Anne Ferguson

Sculptor Anne Ferguson and I are dog-walking mates and as we stroll around the local park keeping an eye on our respective canines, Daisy and Wellington, we often find ourselves swapping notes on shared interests or seeking advice from a kindred spirit on common problems. I have rarely, perhaps never, had a conversation with Anne that has not made me view the world differently. An intensely thoughtful and introspective woman, she has a capacity to analyse issues and shed light on them in a unique way, reflecting a deeply held sense of duty and moral conviction combined with a certain freedom of spirit, a refusal to be bound by conventional concepts and value judgments but insisting on her right as a human being to reach her own conclusions and live her life according to her own carefully thought-through tenets.

When I asked if she would agree to be included in this book her reaction was initially somewhat diffident, asserting that she was too low-profile, too 'ordinary', to be of interest to the world at large. But there was no doubt in my mind not only that as an artist she would add a valuable dimension to the book but also that her contribution would be one that others would find compelling.

Anne's home base is in Mosman in Sydney, where she has lived for virtually all of her adult life and marriage to her lawyer husband, David. I visited her on a hazy morning when the stunning view through the Heads disclosed a still, glassy sea drained of its normal deep blue and merging with the sky so that they appeared as virtually one. I commented that I found such grey days a little oppressive and drab, a view vigorously disputed by Anne who said that she liked these days best of all when the picture was filled with gold and lilac. Suddenly it sprang to life for me too and I wondered how I could ever have seen only a monotone.

Anne's is an old home that has settled comfortably into itself. Deep sofas on dull polished floors combine with mellowed wood tables and chairs, glowing in the soft light. But, as well, the recent renovations which she says provided a metaphor for her life on reaching the fifties and which, at the time, she found difficult to come to terms with, have turned it into a light-filled personal gallery, the white-painted walls and raked glass skylights providing the perfect setting for the wonderful paintings and sculptures in every room.

A few weeks before our meeting I had been to an exhibition of Anne's work and was quite unprepared for the sheer beauty of what she had produced. The smallish-sized sculptures were pieces of exquisite delicacy, shimmering with gold and silver. In another room, pieces of marble, ebony and jade had been carved into sensuous curves begging a caress. Anne has much of significance to say through her art, but she is concerned as well with aesthetic appeal, a view which does not always accord with prevailing philosophies in the art world. She told me that she had received several phone calls from other artists objecting to the fact that her pieces were beautiful as well as expressive.

Anne has had six solo exhibitions of her work as well as participating in numerous group exhibitions. Represented in several major collections, she has also produced many works on commission, including a steel and glass sculpture for Macquarie University and the bronze gates for St Peters Church, Cremorne. Other major commissions include four marble finials for the grand staircase in the new Parliament House, Canberra, and in collaboration with sculptor Peter Corlett, a black granite carving for the Returned Soldiers League memorial.

It was interesting to learn of the difficulties of Anne's early years and the fact that she and her sister were both discouraged from studying art. Not only has Anne been successful as a sculptor and artist, but her sister, Judy

Cotton, who now lives in New York, has also recently had a highly acclaimed exhibition in that toughest of all cities and has had one of her paintings bought by the Metropolitan Museum of Art for hanging in that august gallery.

Anne Ferguson's life is a text-book example of that led by many women of her generation. Married in her early twenties, she gave up work because it was expected. The birth of three children in five years led her to wonder if she could maintain her sanity. It was not until her children were substantially grown that she was free to take some time to further her own artistic development and leave the family for a few months while she studied overseas. It is only now, when family demands have largely been fulfilled that she can concentrate on her own career. She is revelling in her freedom and at a time when many people are thinking of retirement, Anne says the thing that motivates her is 'work, work, work'.

During one of our morning perambulations, unrelated to this book, Anne had said to me that turning fifty had been a real milestone in her life and that on her last birthday, when she reached fifty-five, she had thought long and hard about what it meant. She said she had decided it was rather like a lizard which has its tough, hard skin on the top and then when you turned it over there was the soft white underbelly. The two sides were completely different and that is how she visualised the fifties. She didn't know which side was which, but life before and after fifty was just completely different and what you learned as you progressed through the decade was that you have to go ahead carrying both sides. It was a striking image.

❖ ❖ ❖

I was born in Broken Hill and when I was five we moved to the mountains in New South Wales where my father had a sawmill. I was very badly cross-eyed, my eyes used to roll around like marbles, and there was a man in Orange who said they could fix my eyes with exercises so, when I was six and my sister was four, we were sent to boarding school in Orange. That was not good, it was not a good time. And they didn't fix my eyes. Eventually a young English doctor came who said, what is this nonsense, and he did an operation which was successful so I went home to the country for several more years at a wonderful one-teacher country school. The school was run as a parliamentary democracy by this young man, who I thought was about 105 — he must have been about twenty-three! — and that was a really magical time.

The boarding school at Orange was akin to a Dickensian school and the time there was very difficult. It was very isolating. Being badly cross-eyed means that you have got a physical defect that makes people flinch away, they don't want to look at you, they can't look at you, and I think that the loner quality I have came from there, but also a certain resilience.

When we were ten and twelve we went away to boarding school again because there was no school in that small country town. We went to school in Bathurst which I didn't care for and it wasn't the best education in the world. However, there was a terrific art education which my sister and I both enjoyed, and a good musical education which has also stood us in good stead. Apart from that, I got a passionate hatred of ball games.

In other respects it was a fairly rigid upbringing. We couldn't leave the school grounds, we would see our parents once a term and then we would go home in the school holidays. My parents were hard working, they never took weekends off. I didn't know what a weekend was until I went to boarding school the second time. Then they bought a farm out of town, which was marvellous and from then on we had a wonderful time on holidays and I, because there was nothing else to do, did really well at school and won a scholarship to university. I wanted desperately to go to art school but that wasn't considered to be a good idea.

Looking at it from my parents' perspective, their view was understandable. They had not much money, I had a scholarship, art school was full of this terrible stuff, people you couldn't trust, and what was the use of it anyway, there was no future. So I went to university and I failed everything, the lot. I hadn't got a clue what they were talking about. I had learned by rote everything that was necessary in school and I had never learned to study. I had no idea how you actually studied.

When I failed there was really no future. I couldn't go back to a small country town, there was nothing there, so I did a secretarial course, which I didn't like, I couldn't spell. I got a job in David Jones in the advertising department, because that was close to art, and I went to the Julian Ashton Art School. Thinking back on it, it was amazing. Julian Ashton was full of everybody, all the people who are names now and there I was, seventeen or eighteen, from the country, trying to work out what I was doing and trying to avoid being the model for the group.

I had come to Sydney with a hand-drawn map of the city. I used to get on the bus and ask, which way is the Quay, and try and work out how to get myself around. I didn't have anywhere to live so I got one room in a house with a couple of Christian Scientists who were very kind to me. I had a bedroom and I shared my meals with them and I was really very happy. I read the whole of the Double Bay library because I didn't have any friends. I didn't know anybody, I had lost my university friends, I knew almost nobody in Sydney so I just went to the Double Bay library and read.

I read the United Nations report on Hungary. I thought, this is appalling, this can't be happening, fix it. I know what I'll do, I'll join a political party and fix it. Having had a Liberal background, I joined the local branch of the Liberal Party. [Anne's father, Sir Robert Cotton, had a distinguished career as Liberal cabinet minister and ambassador to Washington under the Fraser and Hawke governments.] After the first meeting I went for a cup of coffee with the oldest man I had ever seen. He was actually my husband-to-be and he is only four years older than I am!

A couple of years later, without my ever leaving the secretarial life but still trying to do some art at night-time at Julian Ashton, I got married. I gave up work, which was an amazing thing to do because we had no money. Of course, it was a great theory at the time that the husband should support you. So there I was with two towels, no money, in a house that we were minding for somebody, because it saved us rent, with a French maid and an Italian gardener and a cage full of birds. I don't know what I did, I have no idea what I did. I think I just learned how to manage. I had never learned before because I had been at boarding school. The French maid taught me to cook. She had a glass, a little kitchen glass, and she would measure everything in the glass. So when we moved to yet another house which saved us rent I couldn't cook because I didn't have the glass and I couldn't remember the measurements.

It was hard, but we managed to save up and buy a small timber cottage in Balgowlah. I got pregnant and I was terribly ill. I gave up art altogether. Then we bought this house that we still live in which was very, very derelict. At that stage we had two children and then we had a third child. So there I was with a five-year-old, a three-year-old and a baby and that was full on. It was just swamp material.

Those years were terrible, although I enjoyed being a mother very much. I did marvellous things with them, lots of very creative things, made kites, did all sorts of things with them. We had a very close relationship but by the time I was twenty-seven I had three small children and I hadn't achieved anything except failure. I had no idea of an identity, I was just rather like a somnambulant. I feel like that time was a sleepwalking time. The twenties were asleep. I was starting to wake up in my teens and suddenly *wham*, what with society and the biological urge, the breeding instinct, I just crashed. So those years, that decade, was a breeding time. I often wonder if women go into almost a psychological shutdown to breed, but that can't be true because women having children later don't do it. It is probably more likely that we were victims of a particularly strong series of social pressures and the only way for us to survive was to close off part of ourselves. Anyway, I had a third child and I thought I was going to go nuts.

So I enrolled in art school. They said, you can do drawing or you can do composition or you can do 3-D. And I said, what is 3-D? And they said, sculpture and it is taught by a man called Bim Hilder, who proved to be the son of JJ Hilder whose work I had known and admired very much. So I said, I'll do 3-D. I had to go Crows Nest Tech one night a week and that's what I did for about four years. I used to draw other people's children in the daytime to help pay for the fees and the babysitting. I went one night a week and it was suddenly the right thing. I didn't actually learn to draw or paint. I couldn't afford it and I didn't have the time.

Then I thought, well, I am not going to be able to have a technical college training the way art students can, so what I am going to have to do is find highly skilled people and learn from them, short and hard. So I did. I found a ceramicist, a potter, to teach me. After that I did a CIG welding course, got someone to teach me bronze casting. It just grew like that.

I don't know why I was so determined, except that I had been put off so many times and the urge was so strong. I don't know why it is so strong but it is in both my sister and myself. She was also refused art training and given the chance at university and she also failed.

There was a wonderful girl who lived next door, who would hop over the fence with her tea on a tray and bath and feed the kids. She has become my best collector. She lives in America now and she has a historical review of my work, that I have never seen, because she and her husband have bought it for years. I would love to see what she has because there it is, a complete review of where it has been and where it is going and where it is at.

I had a studio underneath the house. There was a room, which was very damp but it was empty so I used it. I put in a workbench and worked there while the children were young. The children would come home from school and say, 'What sort of a mood is she in?' I cooked up hot wax on the kitchen stove and blew things up and just generally did what I could, given the confines.

Then a local man called Lindsay Robertson died, very young. They wanted a memorial for him in the Mosman Infants School and they asked if I would make it. He was the landscape architect for the whole of the New South Wales coast and he and I had known each other since school in Bathurst, so we were old, old friends and I was very fond of him. I decided that I needed something strong, that would withstand the depredations of the public and children and all that so I would make it in granite. I didn't have a clue how you worked granite, I had never done it. So I rang a friend in the country who works in granite, she told me how to do it and eventually I made this carving which is still there. The children have climbed on it and it has lasted, the patina is wonderful, really fantastic. It is a good memorial for him, it's small enough for the children to climb and slide on, it has little finger places for them, and it will always be there.

Stone carving came from that. I just went on doing it and one day I was down in the country with my friend, at Easter time. There was a group of sculptors, just friends, having lunch and she said, 'Oh, by the way, this letter's come, they want someone to go to Japan, someone who can carve granite, why don't you go?' I said, 'But I can't go, I have one daughter at university and one doing her higher school certificate and one who is only twelve, how can I go to Japan for three months?' I had another marvellous woman friend who had cancer, who has subsequently died, and I talked to her and she said, 'You have worked a long time,' — by then it was about fifteen years — 'and you have worked very hard and you either take this chance and go on or you stay where you are for ever.' So I went. I was so scared, I had a bad back, I had a back brace on, and I had all my tools because I didn't trust them to supply what I wanted. I didn't know where I was going, I couldn't find it on the map and I went from here in Mosman to Tokyo overnight. I can't believe it now. I had been sent a book, with all these photographs and examples of their work. There were three people from America, one from Australia, one from England, one from Holland, one from Germany, one from Switzerland, one from Russia, and the rest were all Japanese. It was a big park south of Japan, just off the island of Kyūshū. I caught the plane, got a train across from Narita, I had never been to Tokyo, never done any of that before. We were standing in a queue for the bus from Ogori to Hagi and there was a western person behind me, who proved to be one of the people I worked with, and he said to me, 'You're very brave coming to this, you're a woman.' I thought, oh my God!

I lived and worked with them for three months using a common bathhouse. We made a great big granite park out of 450 tons of granite. By the time I had finished I knew how to work granite, but I didn't know when I went, and they all did. They were terribly macho. I said to them once, 'I can't cope with this, all these black egos flying around like bats.' So I got a Superman poster and put it up in the tent and after that they said, 'Ah, Wonderwoman!' It was absolutely fantastic.

David had to stay home and mind the children, convinced that I had gone into a totally untenable situation. He thought it was crazy but he gave me a return ticket and he supported me enough to say, 'If you want to go, go, and remember that you have got a ticket to come home.' It was the most fantastic thing to do. Knowing he thought it was crazy, every moment of it was crazy, but it wasn't.

I feel like that was a postgraduate course. It taught me how to do things technically, way beyond anything I had done. I became very strong, very physically strong, like a teenager who was weightlifting. I came back with calluses across both hands. The hardest thing was coming back. What do you do in Mosman with biceps and calluses? And everybody wanted me to be the same person again. I nearly went mad, I nearly went nuts. Eventually I calmed down which was a good thing to do because the technical and physical ability I had built was the great trap that a lot of men fall into. I completely shut down as a woman in that time. Completely. Physically, mentally, everything: I became a man for three and a half months. It was just extraordinary. But I couldn't go on like that because you can't go on being a man. Well, you can, but I didn't want to. But it took about double the time to readjust.

In the process of readjusting I thought a great deal about what we had done. It was very tough, very aggressive, very geometric, very beautiful, in this park beside the sea which had been a rubbish dump and now had these beautiful pieces of triangular geometry in it which came out of a universal collaboration. Which is what we had. We had a collaboration of different nationalities, cultures, genders, backgrounds and so you get geometry, but I kept thinking, this is the emperor's new clothes. When we laid the last stone in a piece I designed and made with the Dutch man and two Japanese, which was a twenty-metre jetty into the sea, I laid in a Japanese poem and a butterfly's wing from the summer because we went from late summer to winter when it was snowing. We laid it into the concrete and I realised that there was this other side that had not been addressed and that I, as the only woman, had not managed in any way to affect the design and execution of this work. No way.

Another friend, an American sculptor I had talked to before I went, had said to me, 'Don't go, they'll destroy you. You have a western Christian ethic, they have an opposite ethic, they will destroy you.' They didn't, and she then invited me to apply for a course called Yaddo. So two years later I went to Yaddo which is in upper New York State and is the absolute other side of the coin. It is a great castle in Saratoga Springs with three lakes and little castles in the lakes for musicians, with glass windows looking out. It is available for writers, artists and musicians. We were given a studio, accommodation, silence all day. Nobody can contact you, only in dire emergencies can anyone get in touch with you. There are very low numbers and you have to be invited, you can't apply. People like Carson McCullers were there, Edgar Allan Poe wrote 'The Raven' there. It is the most magical place and it was there that I started to address the issues which were in the butterfly and the poem under the stone and that's the other side of the work I do now.

My creative expression is changing as I get older. I am technically very able now, which in a sense worries me. Also, I have much greater courage to do what I regard as female skills. I went to Yaddo to do all this smart stuff. Two days after I got there, I raced into town and bought a bag of plaster. But the real thing that happened was that I started to stitch paper and I realised the moment I put the needle through the paper that I had made an incredibly powerful statement. I couldn't believe the feeling I had of the weight of history behind me. At first I thought I was expressing how I felt tied down. With the first pieces, I felt quite sorry for myself and I thought, this is the Gulliver syndrome and I am tied down by domestic stuff. But over time as I got older I realised it is nothing to do with that, it's to do with the fantastic linking and connections that women have made through time and still continue to make. It is to do with the very fragile, incredibly strong fabric that is still in the Egyptian museums just as the great artefacts are, the fact that Middle-Eastern women are valued for their memories of the patterns, the fact that the cat's cradle is the beginning of mathematics. When I put a needle through the paper, for me it is much more powerful than a chisel.

Now there are two sides to my work. There is the very strong stone-carving side and this very strong ephemeral landscape side. I get a great deal of advice to give up one or the other, but they both inform each other and I can't make one without the other. I can't explain it. I just know that they need to be together to go ahead. Maybe in time that will change. Maybe in time I will get it together. But it is those two sorts of work that seem to me to be the two sides of making value judgments. Through the male stone carving I can express lots of things that I regard as very important that I can't express otherwise. The other side is the secret history of the world that every woman knows and they don't often know they know it. And it is very dangerous to talk about it, we've all been put down for talking about it. This is the first time I have really talked about it.

As a woman artist you feel envious of women without children because they don't face the dichotomy between work and family. Yet you know they also don't have a very deep feeling that you have, an inner knowledge which is almost impossible to tap. I haven't been able to articulate it and I can't work out whether it's a Pollyanna justification for the lack of time or if it is real. But real or not, it is a terrible conflict. The essential feeling for artists is that you must devote your whole life to your work and it doesn't matter what suffers. Other people and other things should suffer or you're not a proper artist. Very few women are willing to do that. Does that make us lesser or does that make the whole value judgment that men have imposed over the centuries, suspect?

Because males have done most things, written, made music, made art, made buildings, made politics, made structures of government, they have worked out what is good, what is excellent. If women have not been involved, even to fifty per cent, how do we know that they are right? I question even my own value judgments because they are coming out of a male structure of what is right and there has been half the world that has not said, yes, this is right for us too.

I don't go along with the theory that women's creativity is blunted by the fact that they have children, that it is expressed by creating a child. I think it is quite the reverse, but it appears and is perceived to be blunted because you are taking the value judgment which doesn't value the other part of their life which they are bringing to their work. For centuries that has not been valued and now, for the first time, we can look at the possibility that that other part of their life is equal or even more valuable in what they create.

Whilst that is changing, it is not fast enough. I think it is the real and serious issue ahead of us, that what is seen to be right is not necessarily so. It needs to be questioned.

The most striking thing about being in your fifties is being able to see the past and the future. There is a moment when you stop. It is almost as though you are given the time to stop and see where you come from, what the future possibly holds. You can't re-invent the past but you can possibly invent the future. It is a very great privilege. I didn't realise that is what would come. I think it goes through to perhaps your late fifties or early sixties when you turn ahead again and go forward. It is not marking time but it is a watershed where you are yourself as much as you can be. You know it is perfectly useless trying to change yourself and, what's more, you are not interested. You no longer have that ghastly feeling of when you're young and you think, I've got to be this, I've got to be tall and blonde, I've got to be ... anything. You don't have to be anyone but yourself now.

We are at the cutting edge. What we are laying down now will be the first time in lots of cases. We are a very privileged generation. We were given the pill. Freedom is in the hands of the drug companies really. If they withdraw it because of some unilateral power then all of these things that we have gained will go backwards. Some women are already going backwards and we have to take that into account. In lots of countries they don't have ready access to birth control, they don't have this ability to look forward. So what we do is terribly important because it may be the base not just for us but for lots of other women in the world who are a long way back.

I think you turn in your sixties. You turn towards something which seems to me very exciting. I don't know what it is but I feel that there is ahead a great discovery of peace. That also comes to you in your fifties, a peacefulness. I think it is to do with the fact that you start to let go, you let go of a lot of responsibilities for the things you can't change. You tend to hand over to people their responsibility for themselves and that is an enormous freedom. Especially the handing over to your children of the responsibility for themselves. Sure, you care for them, and try to be a help, but you are not responsible any more.

What you have trouble with sometimes is making them let you let them go. I feel that if you hang on to your children they will break your fingers. If you hang on long enough, that is what will happen. But also, if they hang on to you long enough you will have a lot of trouble getting them to let you go. It can be a conflict, depending on the particular personalities and that I find very difficult. I find it very tricky, not difficult, but tricky, having this new granddaughter because I can see this enmeshment of love coming back: the old problem of how much love do you give and how much responsibility is involved and is it responsibility, or do you think it is responsibility because of your conditioning, can you give it unconditionally and be free? I look forward to the sixties and being able to resolve those issues. I don't think I can do it in an instant, I think I have to work through it. But just even raising the question within yourself often means there is an answer. The other thing is that things sometimes don't get resolved and you learn, now, that an unresolved question is often dealt with simply by being looked at. You don't have to have the answer and you learn that not having the answer is often the answer itself.

We renovated the house a few years ago and it was quite sad. I was upset that the past was going and I couldn't control what the future held. I was in my early fifties and that's when I started dealing with the issues of the fifties. A lot of walls were knocked down and I felt very unsteady and very unstable. We were out of the place for two years, we were sort of 'unplaced'. It was a very good metaphor for the fifties.

My motivating forces now are work, work, work. At this age it is possible to set out a pattern in your days. At earlier times bits of your day were given over to other things — picking up the children from school, the groceries ... I used to have to work like mad from 9.30 to 3, now it's an extended time. Now there is a great space in your head because you have absolved yourself from lots of responsibility. You don't have to do dinner parties, you don't have to get your toenails painted, you don't have to do any of that stuff which you used to think was important. The fact that you didn't do it mattered. Now it doesn't matter and you know it doesn't matter. It's great.

Society's attitude to older women is disastrous. Absolutely disastrous. It's a real horror. I have some role models who are terrific. There is a woman in her mid-sixties now in America with a fine mind and a very articulate pen, and my friend in her seventies who never stops and who is unbelievably resilient — and frail. They are regarded as outside the norm, but I know they are not. There are these phenomenal women out there but society doesn't recognise or value them.

Why do we live longer than men? We have been given this extra time for a very good reason because we lost time in our twenties when we were somnambulant. We get another ten years and that carries enormous responsibility with it. I don't think society is allowing those women to take up their responsibilities. Why can't you have sixty and seventy-year-old women in parliament? Why do they all have to be twenty-two or thirty-two? It's not real, it's not looking at a resource and using it. The people that I admire almost without exception are older women and if I admire them and if I learn from them, why doesn't society? Why are they typecast and not given the chance?

They have wisdom and tolerance and surely that is invaluable. There is this terrible image of the sort of ga-ga woman with a shopping trolley. There is a lovely lady I know who has got very, very bad arthritis and she has got a walking stick which somebody made for me to measure stone and I gave her. She never measured stone with it but she was shopping the other day and a young man with his mobile phone raced ahead of her into the queue waiting for a taxi and she said, 'Look, I think you've made a mistake, it's my taxi.' 'Oh, I'm very busy and I've got to get to town.' She said, 'I am a very old lady, I have to take my shopping home and if you don't get out of the way, I am going to hit you with my walking stick.' That's what I think of old ladies, I think they're terrific!

I think there needs to be some kind of political activity. The existing structures like the Women's Electoral Lobby don't allow them a voice. How can they? They perceive older women the same way as everybody else. Young women do not see that the future is ahead of them as well. They are not looking to where they will be, not looking to their responsibilities. Perhaps they are just not listening. Why don't we face it? Are we frightened of the future? We push it aside, we pretend it's not going to happen or it is not going to happen to us.

I think our generation is more articulate and will be more able to stand up for themselves. If you look at previous generations you have got women whose health care was not as good as ours, whose education was not as good as ours, whose awareness wasn't as developed as ours. I look at a friend in America who had a very fine education and she is able to still use it. Women's education in Australia was appalling so what you are seeing if you are looking twenty years ahead of us is appalling education, and therefore no resources in the women themselves because their education wasn't up to it. That doesn't apply to everyone. Look at Leonie Kramer. She doesn't have a problem because she has an education, she has a power base to work from, she is able. How much you then enable other women is your responsibility. If you are in that position then your responsibility is perhaps to enable other women to reach that position.

I feel very strongly about that, I feel very strongly about women who are in the grip of a fundamentalist or dictatorial regime either in their own home or in another country. They have to have at least some vision that it is possible to go on growing, that you can offer back to the world what you feel you have to offer. Everybody surely has a right to offer back to the community what is of value to them. If half of the world is silenced, then you must lose; you must lose a very important aspect of how the world can go. If, as people say, the world is in trouble and ecologically endangered, then a gentler touch, a needle, rather than a chisel, is going to be better.

I think ageing is much harder for men. Men find it very hard because the diminution of physical strength for them must be a fearful thought. Also, if they have been powerful in other ways, the loss of that power to which they must obviously become addicted is hard to face. They face the loss of either physical power, strength, or some other way of using power. It must be very frightening for most men unless they are very aware and unless they have looked after a part of themselves which can come with them into a more universal sphere of activity than the God-given right to rule.

I am sure women in particular re-define success as we get older. I have always been very interested in the philosophy of failure because I failed early on. I recently read a marvellous article about the artist Ian Fairweather which defined success on different cultural parameters and said that it is to do with being professional or amateur, which is the Chinese way of looking at painters and is absolutely the opposite of the Western way. The professional for us is the most successful and able person and the amateur is not quite that. For the Chinese artist, and their whole sociological structure, the amateur is someone who is always trying to achieve something that is beyond them. The professional is someone who is satisfied with where they are at. I think we re-define ourselves, because women are trying to achieve something beyond themselves, to go ahead, and often men are satisfied with where they are at. If men are going to go ahead, then they have to start re-defining themselves and what they see ahead of them because they cannot achieve at the same rate as they have before.

I have been married now for nearly thirty-five years. David has been very supportive and I give him full credit for that. He has been very supportive of something he doesn't actually like very much. He is not visually oriented, he doesn't enjoy art very much and it is certainly not something he would do. He would never look at a painting given half a chance. I can move paintings around the house, take them down and sell them and he doesn't know they are gone. Even if I give one to him for his birthday, then I take it away and sell it, forgetting totally that it was a present, he doesn't notice.

In the early days when I went to the tech he came home early, he helped babysit the kids. It was very hard for him because the work was harder and harder to comprehend and the 'why' is very hard to comprehend. But he never questioned the need. He just questioned the directions and he is a very fierce critic because, as a lawyer, his training is criticism. As I watched him try to struggle with what I was dealing with and find areas he just couldn't comprehend it taught me that the public doesn't matter. It is a terrifically hard lesson that you can't expect any feedback, there is none. You do it for yourself or you don't do it.

David is intelligent enough to know, probably before I knew, where I was likely to go and he felt that unless he gave me space to do it I wouldn't stay. Whether he did it consciously or unconsciously he has been very good about it. He hasn't necessarily been supportive in the normal sense that you would expect and often he has appeared to be quite the opposite but I must have a very dogged streak and he has read that. We don't interfere in each other's areas. He very seldom comes to the studio. He came to my last exhibition having not seen any of the work.

It is not necessary that he knows what I am doing. It is not necessary that I know what he is doing. I couldn't understand it and a lot of it he couldn't discuss with me anyway. I learned very early that his work was for him a very creative process that I didn't understand in the slightest degree. I think he has done a terrific job with what he is doing and it makes him happy. So long as he doesn't expect me to go sailing with him too often.

In the end you have a responsibility to do the best job you can in the situation. My daughter says I just believe in marriage. There is a caring for each other that comes out of many, many years and much experience, and terrible ups and terrible downs, a support structure. It is not always based on understanding and it doesn't have to be. It is a difficult issue. I don't understand why marriages last beyond one day. Perhaps it's like an alcoholic, each day at a time.

Getting older doesn't worry me in the least. I worry sometimes about ill health but I don't expect it so therefore I don't dread it. I expect that I have to take care of my health, that it is not a given, but my main worry is that I will have accidents, monstrous accidents at work. That worries me. I worry about the time I can no longer carve stone. But then I have this marvellous friend who is carving granite and she is seventy-three and she has just had a new hip and a new knee, she's planning to have another new knee this year, and she is finishing a ten-pound block of granite. So why should I dread anything? I feel you do it, whatever you are going to do you do, and hopefully there will be this opening-out of understanding where you understand better what your work has been telling you. You understand more clearly the path ahead. Hopefully you won't have too many demands on you to interfere with where you want to go and anyway you will be old enough and sane enough to balance them. I am frightened of too many demands on me, that's my real fear of getting older, not getting older per se but other people demanding of me time I haven't got a lot of. Time is always the really important issue. Especially re the family. If love is anything it is responsibility and that is a problem timewise.

Ageing parents is my big fear. It's really hard. My brother is going off to America and my sister is in America so my parents are used to having a bigger family than just me to support them. They will need an enormous amount of physical time in the next little while and obviously there is more ahead. I don't know how to allocate it. I'll have to learn. I can't expect anyone to do it for me. I keep thrashing around inside my head thinking, who can I ask how to do this? There has got to be an answer, and there isn't. I know there is no answer and there is nowhere to look but I will have to work it out and remember what I have learned, because otherwise I will be subsumed into the demands that automatically happen. The demands will happen because I love them dearly and I can't let them battle on their own and because they are fun. It's not even a guilt trip or any of those things but it does need time, twenty-four hours a day basically, and it can't be available. That is my big fear. How to learn to deal with it, how to balance it. There has got to be a magic answer somewhere.

I have one very, very unfulfilled dream: I am going to go back to the country and live there. It's a fantasy. I have a lot of unfulfilled dreams and what I learned was that they didn't have to be fulfilled because I could always make them. That's what I do in the studio, I make them. I have learned that there is no perfect place unless I make it. But I have this great unfulfilled dream that I will no longer have to live in the city and I will return to the country and it will be as it was when I was a child. I keep finding places. I found this wonderful old church in the country but I don't know. I will probably just keep working.

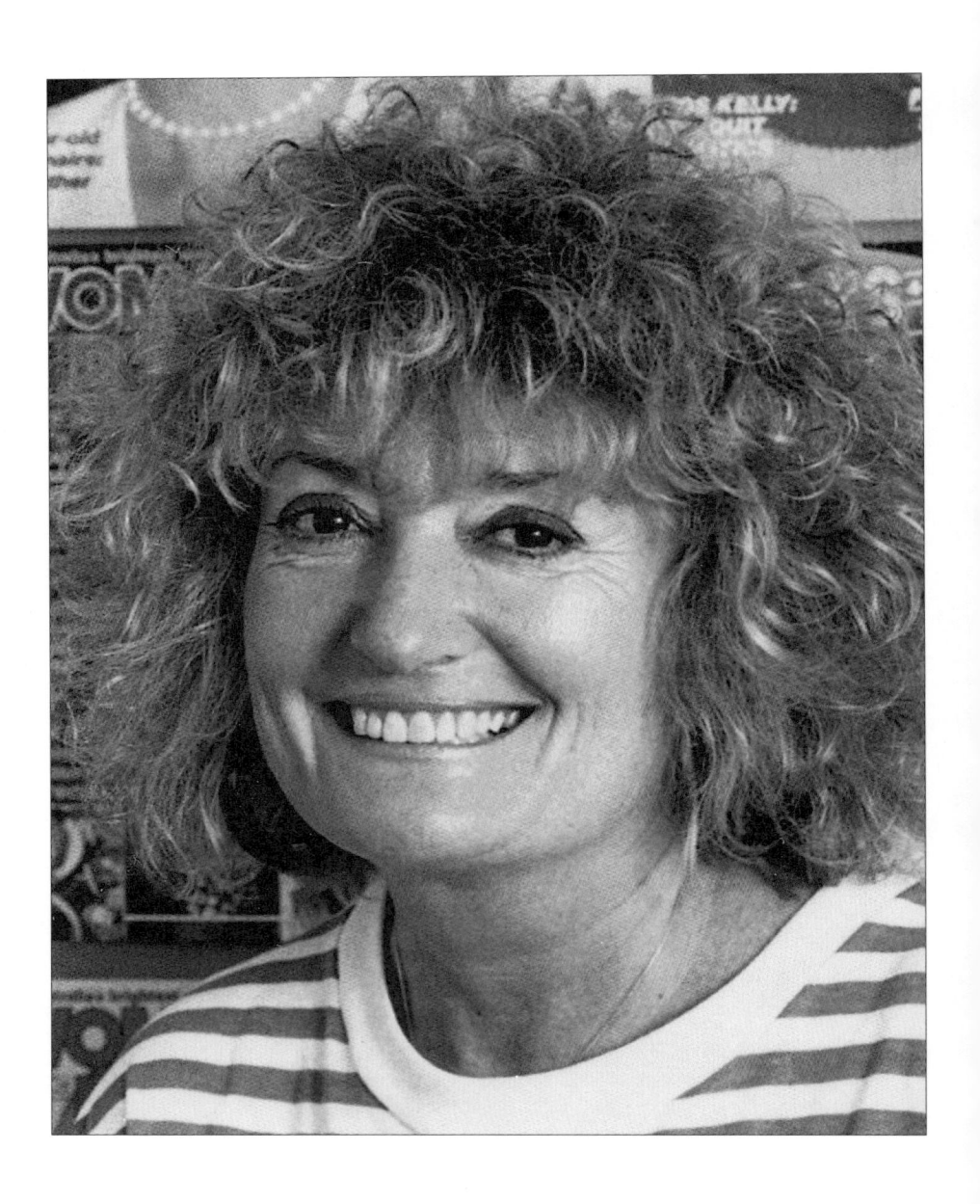

*I think I have reached the stage where I realise how lucky I am and that
I have had this wonderful time in my life, been in the right place at the right
time, made it work.*

❖ ❖ ❖

Nene King

Nene King has been described as the most powerful woman in Australia. As the guiding force behind the two biggest-selling magazines in the country, the description cannot be dismissed as mere hyperbole. First she steered *Woman's Day* from about fourth in circulation to being the top-selling magazine in Australia, selling more than one million copies a week, and then an ecstatic Australian Consolidated Press persuaded her to take on the added burden of the *Australian Women's Weekly*, already the top-selling monthly. The 'Nene King' magazines had a combined readership of more than six million a month. That can reasonably be described as power.

Then, at the age of fifty-one and at what seemed to be the crest of a very large wave indeed, Nene stunned everyone by resigning. She said she was tired, she had no time for the people she loved and, in general, life seemed hardly worth living. At first, no one believed it. Then they thought there must be some hidden agenda. But there wasn't. Hidden agendas aren't part of Nene King's make-up. It was really true that this most upfront of people had simply had enough. She wanted out so she got out and couldn't understand what all the fuss was about.

She didn't stay out for long, it is true. She left ACP with an open invitation to return if ever she changed her mind and, perhaps not surprisingly, after a time she did miss the stimulation of the magazine world and so she took up the offer — but this time, on her terms. She has no intention of getting on the treadmill of exhaustion again.

With her strong square face, liquid brown eyes and tousled mop of blonde hair, Nene King is an irresistible personality. Warm, expansive, feisty, generous of spirit, and totally without pretension, she meets life full on. Everything about her seems to make a statement — her clothes, her gestures, her intense joie de vivre. This is a woman whose passions run unashamedly deep but, at the same time, like a mildly active volcano, bubble constantly to the surface, their owner revelling in the intensity of the life-experience.

I went to Nene's attractive Victorian-era home in a pleasant but unostentatious neighbourhood one sunny morning in late winter. The well-established trees lining the streets were responding to unseasonal warmth by bursting into early bud and neighbours were deferring chores in favour of a chat over the fence on such a lovely day. It was a peaceful scene typifying any one of a number of Sydney suburbs and presumably peopled, both inside and outside the modest houses, with her readers.

My ring at the doorbell brought a cacophony of animal sounds and, on entering, a rumbustious welcome from a pair of dogs. Nene's attempt at discipline was relievedly abandoned when I assured her that I had a much-loved dog of my own and that I (and my clothes) were well-used to such assaults. Once inside the living room, it was possible to observe a cat asleep in a deep chair. What didn't become evident until later was that there was another cat behind another chair, and still another cat on its bed behind the heater. Animals play a large part in Nene's life.

Nene's house is a delightful jumble of a busy life. Books, bowls of fruit, deep comfortable chairs and a vast collection of bric-à-brac reflect a desire to embrace and absorb as many interests and experiences as possible.

Before we could begin our talk, Nene was concerned to ensure the comfort of her visiting father, that he was not too hot or too cold, that he should feel free to turn on the television, that he didn't feel excluded from the living area of the house. A charming man, clearly as devoted to his daughter as she is to him, he had warned me early on that I would have to compete with the telephone, and it proved to be so. At this stage of her life, Nene might have opted out of the hurly-burly of working life but the office mountain was obviously prepared to come to Mahomet. Our talk was frequently put on hold while she dealt with some query or other or issued instructions to erstwhile colleagues. She was clearly being missed.

Like so many other women, in her fifties Nene seems to have got her life together for the first time. So often it is assumed that highly successful women have led a charmed existence and it was sobering to learn that at thirty, she was totally adrift. Many of us will identify with that. Perhaps it is the strength needed to fight back from rock-bottom personal despair that leads eventually to the ability to overcome other obstacles and forge a path in the broader workplace environment.

Nene's decision to 'downstep' is one that other women who have climbed to the top of the corporate ladder are choosing in increasing numbers. There is perhaps an irony that many women complain about the existence of the glass ceiling, the fact that making it beyond a certain level of seniority is still an opportunity denied them, while women such as Nene who do make it, find when they get there that the price is too high, that fourteen-hour days, no family life and the increased risk of dropping dead in their prime are not worth the rewards of mere money and status. Other women are frequently the most strident critics of those who take such a step. It is letting other women down, they cry, reinforcing the male view that women don't have what it takes, that they can't hack the pace, don't take their careers as seriously as men. But it takes considerable courage to opt out, to say, well, there it is, I've got there and I don't like it. Money and status are not easy to give up, for anyone, and Nene's decision may give other senior executives, male and female, cause to pause and take stock, to re-evaluate their lives and ask themselves what life is really all about.

❖ ❖ ❖

I was born and raised in Melbourne, in a very traditional comfortable lifestyle and also I was born and raised a Jew which probably is important if you look at what happened in my life. I went to the Methodist Ladies' College. I did very well at school, although I hated it. I finished school at a very early age, at sixteen, and nobody knew what to do with me. I certainly didn't know what I wanted to do, all I wanted was to have a party. So my mother took me on the 'grand tour' for six months. Then I came back and because my brother had just finished law at

Melbourne University and the books were still around they said, okay, Nene, you had better go off to university and study law too. I did and I hated it. I hated it because I had been regimented all my life with study and suddenly I had freedom and it was most unsuccessful. I need to be regimented, even now I could never freelance. So that first year didn't work out and a friend of my brother's, Michael Schildberger, said to me, why don't you come and have a look at journalism.

I became a reporter at Channel Nine in Melbourne and worked in the newsroom with Sam Lipsky and Michael Schildberger and Bob Kersey, some wonderful people. They tried me on camera. I think I was the first woman reporter in television but it wasn't very successful. I was nervous on camera so they took me off and I wrote news and then I became the chief of staff. I also worked on a program called *Nightwatch*. I used to hang out of a news car every Saturday night and report on all the terrible things that happened in Melbourne on a Saturday night. People would be dying on the road or being burned to death and I'd have a microphone under their noses. Then I fell in love with a cameraman and followed him to England. It was 1965 and I sailed to England and did the full 1960s bit. I worked in London, lived in Chelsea, stomped around in my big clumpy shoes and was a hippy. We got married in 1967 and went on our honeymoon on the Trans-Siberian Railway, which in those days was very exotic because no one got into Russia, and we made a documentary. I wrote it, he filmed it, we edited it and we sold it to America. They were interested in anything out of Russia. Then we thought, where do we go from here, we don't want to go all the way back to Australia, where can we work, and Hong Kong was it.

I stayed in Hong Kong for three years working on an afternoon newspaper as a reporter covering riots. Then I became the entertainment editor and the women's editor and my marriage fell in a heap, because it was just a wild and woolly place and I was the worst wife in the world.

I became quite ill in Hong Kong, basically because my liver packed up, so I went home to Mum in Melbourne, stayed with her, and tried to get a job on Melbourne newspapers. They didn't want to know about all the wonderful things that I had done overseas so I came to Sydney and got a job on the *Sydney Morning Herald*. As soon as I had a job in Sydney the Melbourne people wanted me. It was extraordinary. You know, look what we have pinched from Sydney!

I stayed with the *Sydney Morning Herald* for only six months. I had just walked in off the street and said, 'Hi, I'm Nene King – this is what I do,' and I was hired. But I wasn't happy in Sydney, I missed my parents. So I got a job on the *Melbourne Sun* — it was the *Sun News Pictorial* in those days — in the Women's

Section. The editor of the Women's Section went on leave to write a book for three months and I did her job. When she came back I went back on to wedding captions. She didn't approve of me and I think she wanted to put me back in my place. I fell in love again around my thirtieth birthday. He was a sports reporter and we were married for about eighteen months. He was very strict. I look at the different stages of my life and if anyone was strict with me now I'd shoot them. I was sort of upstaging him in my career because he thought that Peter was the journalist and Nene was the one who should stay at home. So I pulled out of my job and went to work for my father who in those days had a chain of clothing stores in the western suburbs.

We tried to have children. That didn't work, and I discovered that I wasn't able to have a child. That sent our marriage into a heap because he really should have married a virginal Yugoslav, a younger woman, who could have babies. I was older than him, I wasn't a Catholic, I was Jewish, and I had been married before. The whole thing fell in a heap.

I went into a flat on my own and then my life really crumbled around me. I drifted, I wasn't in journalism, and I was so unhappy. I reached absolute rock-bottom. I was almost suicidal — although I'm afraid of dying, funnily enough. I guess that must have been the turning point. From then on I just respected myself more.

Then I met a wonderful woman journalist called Freda Irving and she said, come and do three days a week at *Woman's Day*, in the bureau in Melbourne, and that was lovely. I had a lot of friends there. But Dulcie Boling was just taking over *New Idea* and I was about the first person she hired. I knew nothing. I never thought about anything except the next day, but she was going to revamp *New Idea*, away from crocheting and knitting and whatever, and I fitted in. I was very news-oriented and I introduced, as we used to say, 'the dumb chums', the animal stories and the showbiz stories, all the things basically that I was interested in. In those days there was not much competition. *Women's Weekly* was the big one, Ita Buttrose was there and she was getting a little more serious, but we came in, this little nothing — I think we were selling 480 000 — and we started to catch up. It was a wonderful relationship between two women for a lot of years.

I stayed with *New Idea* for nearly ten years but I came to the conclusion that I would always be second string. I was the chief reporter, the news editor and the deputy editor and that's where I stayed. After nearly ten years it got too much for me and I just resigned with no prospect at all. I am a real Pisces – instant decisions.

Then – nothing happened! Melbourne was pretty tight and magazines were my forte so I came up to Sydney and hawked myself around. I can remember having breakfast with Richard Walsh and he said, 'Who are you and what do you do?' and I said, 'Well, I've been partly responsible for the success of *New Idea* in the last ten years,' because we knocked off all the other magazines. He looked at me like I had two heads because there were no names on the front of the masthead when I was there, it was just Dulcie, and he said, 'Well, er, ... ' To cut a long story short, then I had lunch with Gil Chalmers who was editing *Woman's Day*. She obviously knew a bit more about me and she offered me the job of deputy editor of *Woman's Day*. That was when Fairfax owned it. Then Kerry Packer bought the Fairfax magazines he wanted like *Dolly* and *Woman's Day*, the ones that had potential. Gil wanted to go back to Queensland to have another baby and I couldn't get her out quickly enough. Virtually the day we moved into Consolidated Press and came under the Packer umbrella I became editor of *Woman's Day*. At last I had the chance to show people what I could do. It was selling about 680 000. I revamped it, I redesigned it, I put in the contents that I wanted and it went through the roof. I picked up about 400 000 buyers a week. I made sure everyone talked about *Woman's Day*, I cross-promoted it, I turned it into a very profitable business. It was making money when I took over but by the time I finished with it, it was making a hell of a lot more money. I hasten to add that that had a lot to do with the wonderful people at ACP and how they directed me, because I am not very good with figures, and they looked after a lot of that side of it. Nevertheless, the editors of *Woman's Day* and *Women's Weekly* were answerable for the profit and loss, the circulation, we had to run each magazine as a business.

I am a typical *Woman's Day/Women's Weekly* reader. *Women's Weekly* was a little harder for me. I am a typical *Woman's Day* reader. I love to watch a soppy mini-series. When I am on holidays I read a trashy book. I love gossip, I am interested in film stars, I love to look at how the other half lives. So I was in tune with the market. People say to me now, Nene, what was the secret of your success? It was not some sort of massive plan that I had, it was purely instinct. I just knew what the market wanted. I didn't give them what I thought they wanted, I gave them what they wanted. Big difference.

I think slinging off at women's magazines in the way some people do is an insult. It's an insult to women because we are not taking a gun to 1.2 million women and saying, you have to buy this magazine, or, you are such a schmuck, you buy that magazine automatically, like a robot. We must be giving them something they like to balance their lives, that they want it every week. I used to dismiss the comments but now I think it's an insult. Also, I believe we have to understand the masses and that they have not had the opportunities, perhaps, that we have had to go to MLC and university or whatever.

Think about AIDS, about breast cancer, about menopause. Where does it get the most reaction? I have read stories about menopause for years and years. What did I do in *Women's Weekly*? I got famous women. I got Maggie Tabberer, Kathryn Greiner, Rowena Wallace and I sat them around with a doctor, Sandra Cabot. I got sacks full of letters from women saying, thank you, thank you, I thought I was going mad. It's the way of the world. We talked about AIDS. Do you know when people really took notice of AIDS? Because of Elizabeth Taylor. They suddenly showed an interest – what is it that this woman is doing? So in a funny sort of a way we have really helped get these very important issues across, like breast cancer and cervical cancer. You can put some sort of really heavy piece into the *Financial Review* or something, and that's fine. But if you want to get to the masses, do it the way I do it. I have analysed this and I have got my line ready for people now. I have instant market research. It is a brown envelope at midday every Friday that shows me my figures. If they didn't like what I was doing or thought I was insulting or lowering the standard or whatever they wouldn't buy me.

People scoff at ELVIS PRESLEY SLEPT WITH HIS MOTHER, or DEMI MOORE'S FAKE BREASTS which of course is just all part of the mix. What tends to be forgotten is that I went to a lot of trouble to get really good people in whatever area I was covering, whether it was health or nutrition or whatever. You have got no idea of the response to our doctor column. There are thousands of women out there who don't want to go to a doctor. They're too embarrassed to go to a doctor but they write to the women's magazines. We have sex problems, you have no idea what comes in. I do believe that apart from entertaining we do inform and provide an extraordinary service. I am not going to sit here and apologise for these magazines. They are part of our culture for better or for worse and I think they have done some wonderful things.

I resigned because I'm vain and I've got an ego and I have watched other women in my position disappear without a trace. I didn't want to do that. I wanted to be a success, I wanted my reputation intact when I resigned. I was also exhausted. Running two massive magazines, I was exhausted and I recognised that. The company said, go off for three months, do what you want to do. I loved the company and I particularly loved Richard Walsh. But I wasn't going to be as strong or as good in my job for much longer. I believe I had the courage to say, you've got to get on with it. I have been able to take a rest and I still believe there is a lot of puff in the old girl and I intend to pass on as much and help as much as I can for the next few years. But I stood back and saw myself and I knew I couldn't continue to work day and night, seven days a week, for much longer. It was killing me.

It was also connected with my third husband, Patrick. He is a diver and he lost a diving buddy, who drowned in front of him. I didn't know the man well, he didn't mean that much to me, but I think late in life I have found true love. Pat and I have been together for nineteen years. We have lived together and we were married last year. The day his buddy drowned was a Sunday and we were going out to lunch with friends. I was just getting up, I had been reading page proofs and I was so tired. Pat rang me and he said, 'I'm going to be late for lunch,' and I said, 'Why?' and he said, 'Paul's just drowned.' I'll never forget it. I just could not believe it, not so much because of Paul, but because of Patrick. I can remember sitting at this guy's funeral and I had never seen Pat upset but he sobbed and I looked at him and I thought, you know, I don't see him and I love him so much. It's a wimpy thing to say but it was the other thing that really changed my life. I thought, I'm going to do something about this and get a life. I was always so tired. I couldn't speak, I was exhausted and I would dread the phone, it would ring in the night, and I would be waiting for the taxi to bring the blueprints, and I had done this for nearly twenty years. I don't know why but I suddenly thought, maybe my time's running out, I've got lots of precious people and I am an absolute horror to live with. I've made a success – and I'm getting out. Getting out of that terrible lifestyle. So that's what I did. I told Richard Walsh. I told him on the Thursday morning when I had had breakfast and he asked me to think about it over the weekend. On the Monday I saw the head of the company and we talked it through and, as everyone knows, it hit the fan. It was a funny thing to happen, with all the publicity and everything. But I have never regretted it. I am glad that I am able to stay in it because I am rested now and I don't think I've got one foot in the grave yet so I am pleased that I can pass on my knowledge. But I am just a different person.

I did take a break. I did go up to Coolum and buy another house but then I thought, well, okay, what do I do now? I still like the idea of being involved in magazines but not the hands-on that I had. What we haven't done is train up people and I quite enjoy that. There are editors there that I hope to be able to help. I am going to lie on the beach and enjoy myself as well. But what I did realise when I had had a holiday and a rest is that I wasn't ready to lie on the beach full time. I am very, very lucky. I don't have a family, I don't have commitments, I can run my own race. I deeply regret not having a family, that was beyond my control. But in some ways because of it I have been able to direct my destiny. The only thing I worry about is who is going to feed the animals when I go away. A lot of people have a lot more strings attached to their lives and I don't. I suppose at this stage I am very lucky financially and personally. I am very happy.

Basically, now I will run the *Women's Weekly* and I will probably help as a consultant on other magazines. I suggested to Richard Walsh that I have a good reputation out there in the marketplace and they should use me when they are dealing with big clients. I am quite good with dealing with clients so it makes sense that I can be more of a PR person out there in the marketplace. I never did that before, I never went anywhere except for a few multi-million-dollar advertising accounts. I enjoy that. I have just come back from Townsville where I judged the fashions on the turf. To me that was just a joy. I've never got out into the country and of course you say *Women's Weekly* out there and it's like royalty. It's just beautiful, I love that. I will pick what I do. I have been invited to talk to business people and to conventions and I won't do that because I wouldn't know what to say. I can tell them how we got rid of someone's chins or changed the colour of Fergie's dress and how I got the Fergie toe-sucking pictures but I can't give them some powerful piece on the strategy and the way I marketed the magazines that became such a success because it was just hit and miss.

I have a contract with the company for a while longer and we'll see how it goes. We have the house in Queensland and we probably will move up there eventually but I don't think we are quite ready just yet to do it full time. I know Patrick isn't. Also, we don't want to sell this house. We would be mad to sell real estate in Sydney at the moment. It's nice to have the freedom of choice. I have been invited to try for a radio program. Someone asked me to write a book but most of the stuff that I would write would be libellous. I have been offered some wonderful television but I am tied to the Nine Network so that clipped my wings a bit. I have just never been in this position before.

In terms of age, turning fifty wasn't an especial milestone in my life. It wasn't any big deal. Because of my hectic lifestyle, and the way I have worked my guts out, and I played hard in my years in London and Hong Kong, I was rather grateful I was still here.

The thing that really concerns me is that you are perceived to be old and you don't feel old. It is not so much that you are fifty as such, but suddenly you say 'fifty' to people and they sort of look at you and you can see them thinking, oh my God, she's in the grave. That's disappointing because you don't feel any different. I've slowed down, my eyesight is wobbly now, I've put on weight and men don't lust after me, but these are just trite little things. I told everybody I was going to ignore fifty. I will probably stay forty-nine forever.

Some interesting things did happen to me though, and I think women should be aware of it. Somebody said I was having a mid-life crisis. But I have always been an up and down sort of person and I think because I was so tired I got very down. When I gave up my job, I was visiting dear friends of mine in Melbourne, whom I had known for many years, and I had a row with them. I can't imagine why, but I was just history, my body was crying out and my hormones were going in all directions. So maybe I did have a mid-life crisis. I don't know. What I admire about me, and about a lot of women I know, is that we stop and think, oh God, I am falling in a heap, something's going wrong, I am going to do something about it. A lot of the time people, men especially, just don't do that. They soldier on, they drink too much, they go off and have an affair with a twenty-year-old and all sorts of things. I am sure that physically and mentally all sorts of things were happening to me but I was lucky enough to realise it and do something about it.

I'm lucky, I have had a lucky life. I have been able to learn from my mistakes. I have been able to pull back and see what is happening to me so in that way I have had a bit of control or not got completely out of control.

Turning thirty was my crisis. The thirties were my worst time. My forties were wonderful. My fifties are turning out to be wonderful too but I am scared that I am running out of time because I have always been very afraid of dying, not of the pain, but I haven't come to terms with what is going to happen. I don't know if there is a next life, if there really is a God, if everyone is together and unless someone can prove that to me I am panic-stricken. I am panic-stricken that I won't have Patrick, I won't have my parents, I won't have my animals. In your fifties, and especially as I am having such a good time and have been for a while, apart from getting exhausted, you think, oh God, time's running out. You do wake up and think, oh dear, a lot of my life's behind me now. I guess in your fifties you try and make the most of what you have got.

The big thing about the fifties, though, is self-confidence. In my twenties I wouldn't be seen outside without my make-up, in my thirties I learned to make love properly ... in my fifties, confidence, that's the big thing.

Patrick is eight years younger than me, he's forty-three. I used to worry that he would go off with a little lassie. When I said, I'm retiring, he said, hang on a minute, what about me, because he is such a clever man. But he has found a true love in his diving so we have separate lives and we come together every so often. He'll go off on a holiday, which is what he is doing now, with a whole lot of friends, and go diving. There have never been any restrictions. We do what we want to do within reason, and then we meet. It's wonderful. The total freedom. I think that is a throwback from my second marriage where I was put under the thumb and I thought, I'll never do this again.

I had plastic surgery when I was thirty. I had my eyes done. I thought I had bags under my eyes and I thought it was the end of the world. I had done a story on this plastic surgeon and he said, 'Nene, if you ever want ...' So at thirty I went and got the bags removed to try and make myself look younger. I had no confidence in myself. I thought I was in love with somebody who didn't like women working and who wanted me to have a baby. I was under a lot of personal pressure, and perhaps that interfered with my thinking, but I said, I'm thirty — my life is over. Really, my life was just beginning.

I actually think about having a face-lift now but first I would try to lose some weight. I am more concerned about it at this stage because now I have seen all the face-lifts that have gone wrong. I have done a lot of stories on them. I wouldn't have a face-lift to keep a man, but if it helped me and gave me confidence I would be off there and having one.

I do nothing to keep fit. I hate exercise. I tried when I started to get really run down with doing the two magazines. I got a personal trainer and I used to exercise three times a week but to me that was such a drag. I would take my clothes into the Hyde Park Club. I had to be there at six o'clock because I started work at half past seven, and I used to dread it. I hate exercising. I eat rubbish, I do nothing to keep fit. I suppose I should, but it's a bit late now.

I have no idea about the future because I have always been a person who hasn't planned things. I hope I live with Patrick for the rest of my life because he is just so wonderful. I must have done something good in another life to have ended up with him. I hope that he stays well and that we're together. I wish I could say how I feel about the future. I don't want to not work so I hope that the opportunities still come along for people to want to use me. I don't want to be seen as a has-been or, you know that silly old Nene King is still hanging in there. In this industry, I look at the youngsters and I'm so old. I shall try and retire gracefully eventually.

I don't have any things I wish I had achieved and I haven't. I think I have reached the stage where I realise how lucky I am and that I have had this wonderful time in my life, been in the right place at the right time, made it work. I am more of a realist now. I used to dream, I used to look at *Woman's Day* and think when I was at *New Idea*, if I had that magazine what I could do with it. My dreams have come true for me, both in my personal life and in my working life. Now I am just hanging in there.

I do think in a lot of areas in the workforce, women stop. They can't go any further. They are kept on the factory floor and that disappoints me. I was the first woman on the Nine Network board and I found that sort of attitude, what's she doing here, what does she know ... It disappoints me that women go so far and that's it. In a funny sort of way, although I have become an editor and an editor-in-chief and all that, I didn't go any further. There are other women in management at ACP but the publisher is always a man. I find that we seem to stop. They just let us go so far and that disappoints me.

I am such a forceful person. I just break down the barriers and prove myself if I want to. As the years went by and my figures were on the board and the sales were good, I used that. Not so much for my personal gain but to get what I wanted to make those magazines better. Then of course you become a bitch. I think the best thing with me, probably because of the way I look or my wonderful relationship, they didn't say I had slept with anybody to get to the top.

There are so many things that I have been so proud of but in general terms my greatest achievement professionally is taking *Woman's Day* from a very lazy number — three or four I think we were — to the number one magazine in Australia. That goes with a wonderful group of people who helped me do it and so it is me and a lot of other people, but in terms of professional achievement I suppose I'll go down as whipping *Woman's Day* along. But also ending up happy. I find it quite extraordinary for the sort of life I've led that I keep getting these chances.

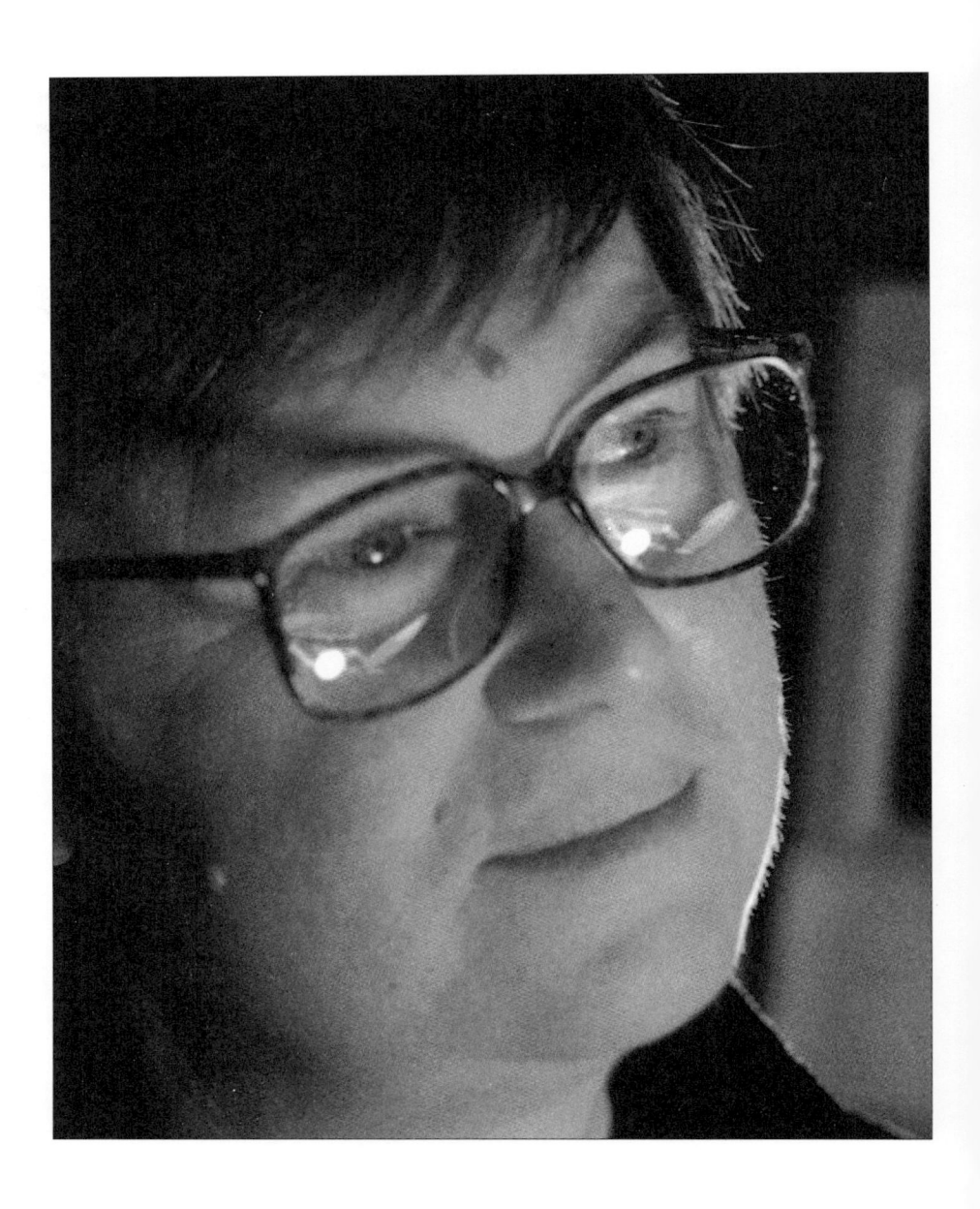

I think that because I have experienced all that I have, all the disjointedness and the sadness and the ups and the downs I have an optimism about being able to do things that a lot of other women my age don't seem to have.

❖ ❖ ❖

Helen Leonard

Helen Leonard was the only woman in this book whom I had not only not met previously but had no prior knowledge of at all. I had asked the Women's Electoral Lobby if they could suggest someone suitable who was not well-known, who did not have a high profile, in other words, someone 'ordinary'.

When I telephoned, her warm voice was immediately appealing and we arranged a preliminary meeting in a small outdoor café, opposite her office. It was a sunny day with a balmy breeze and the scavenging pigeons added to the unpretentiousness of the surroundings. There was an instantaneous rapport. It was impossible not to like this softly spoken, unassuming woman and easy to make a judgment that here was someone who had much of significance to say, with a life that other women would both identify with and find an inspiration in.

At forty-nine, Helen is looking forward to the fifties. She asserts with some humour that she has finally reached the conclusion that women are either good or mad. After years of battling to be a good woman she has now decided she would rather be mad. 'You go mad trying to be good because it is impossible. I didn't ever feel that I was good, I just spent my whole life trying to live up to a dream.'

Helen elected for us to meet again at her home and I presented myself in the early evening, after work, at her small inner-city terrace. Comfortably cluttered, the house is filled at long last with the furniture which had belonged to her mother and which she refused to part with for so long. On a cold night, a warming cup of tea was instantly on the table with home-made biscuits made not, I was informed with considerable feminist satisfaction, by Helen herself but by a young man in the office who has taken it on himself to keep his workmates supplied with tea-break goodies.

Helen's story is one that will strike a chord with many women. Born into circumstances she describes as humble and a product of the era, it did not occur to her that she would do other than marry, have children and be a good and supportive wife and mother. She married the boy who asked her because that was what you did and it saved the money you spent on going out. It was twenty years before she even began to express herself in a way that she found fulfilling. 'Ten years ago I would have thought that I would be in a nice big house surrounded by grandkids. Now what I'm going to do with grandkids is outrageous things. I'm going to teach them to be outrageous, teach them to be themselves.'

Helen's life has had more than its share of sadness and difficulties and the fact that she has risen so far beyond those early horizons with, as she makes clear, comparatively little education and no underlying sense of her place in the world, speaks volumes for her courage and tenacity and refusal to let her life be ruled by external circumstances.

It is interesting that, in the end, her decision to leave her marriage was taken because of her realisation that the family situation was, most of all, damaging her children. An unexpected, albeit ultimately unsuccessful pregnancy was the catalyst in making her assess the relationship and decide that this was not an environment into which a new life could be brought. Many women will identify with that. So often women tolerate intolerable situations when their own wellbeing is the only issue and are driven to take action only when they see that their children are suffering. And yet it is not uncommon for accusations of selfishness to be levelled — how could she break up the children's home? — a gratuitous assumption which invariably overlooks the fact that the formal act of separation is usually merely a public acknowledgment of an event that has taken place in all the ways that are important many years earlier.

Like most women of her time, Helen's main activity outside the home consisted of voluntary work. In fact, she not only was not paid, her activities cost her money, in the sense that she met the (often considerable) expenses incurred. She recounts with some amusement that when she was offered her first paid job, she found it difficult to comprehend and indeed accept that she would receive money for work she had done for nothing for so long.

Helen is now project officer at the New South Wales Office on Ageing, a job which includes taking responsibility for implementing the global radio hook-up for the International Day for the Elderly, in liaison with the United Nations, Radio Australia and ABC networks, commercial and community radio. She also runs the Seniors' Media Training Program, which aims to provide media skills to representatives of major seniors' organisations.

The fit seems perfect. A woman with proven organisational skills, an understanding of how community organisations work and a natural compassion, helping to lead the way for women of her own generation, ensuring that their talents are utilised and their needs are taken account of.

WEL had interpreted my requirements with commendable accuracy. Helen was an ideal subject for this book. She is most certainly not, however, 'ordinary'.

❖ ❖ ❖

My parents were the gardener and the housekeeper for a big property in Pymble and so I grew up very much as the 'gardener's daughter'. I was conscious of class although I didn't know that was what it was. I always felt different and less than everybody around me. The other thing was that Mum and Dad drank a lot so there was always either a lot of love or I didn't exist. They were in a world of their own.

Apart from those things it was a very traditional family. Mum was an excellent housekeeper. She had left home in really bad circumstances in the bush and she went into service when she was thirteen. Our house was kept better than the houses that she worked in – and that included things like manners and the kinds of meals we were served and all those things. Being polite and being nice were very, very important. Because Mum and Dad were who they were and Dad had left school in fourth class and Mum was thirteen when she started working, we didn't know about education. There was a lack of insight and understanding about what education was, although we knew it was important. Mum used to be quite impressed by what she called 'schoolmarms' — she didn't use the word 'teacher', it was always 'schoolmarms' — and she knew that education was important. She had known somebody who had stayed at school until they were eighteen and this was the highest goal to attain. So I went to the local public school and then to the selective high school which was a shock because I didn't understand what 'selective' high schools were.

I couldn't work out how I got there. I used to deliberately do badly because I didn't understand the world. I was in the top sixth class, but I came last in it. I passed everything always, but only just. It was a terribly confusing time because I had no framework to fit any of these things into. Mum sent me off to the selective high school to do typing and shorthand because this is what girls did but of course they didn't do those kinds of things at the high school, they did languages. I struggled on.

When I left school there was no thought at all about going to university which, when I think back, was very unusual because as an academic high, the school was aimed at getting their young women students into university. I went off into nursing.

I loved the caring part of nursing but the world still didn't make sense to me so once I got to the responsible positions it was a real trial. Around that same time I had an accident and hurt my back and ended up in traction for six months. I left nursing and got a job as a dental nurse, and later on as a doctor's receptionist.

My parents' drinking was a real issue for me when I was growing up. There was a family code of secrecy around it. If you put it into the context of the times, you really took notice of what the neighbours thought, so it was very important for any neighbours or friends not to know what really went on behind closed doors. The way that I dealt with it was that as soon as they took their first drink I would put a kind of blank wall around myself and just pretend, just stop the world. I must have done this for a lot of years because by the time I went nursing there was a real gap between me and reality and it took a lot of years to recover. I'd taken a code of, I'm never going to cry, I've got to survive through this, so I dissociated myself from feelings and it took a lot of years to recover all of that afterwards. I think it wasn't until I had children that it came together.

I got married when I was twenty-one. Again, the normal pattern and the socialisation was that you went to school, you did a bit of work and you got married. All my friends had boyfriends and were pairing off. A young man who needed me asked me to marry him and I loved being needed. There was something there we called love and we got engaged. We were always strapped for money and we decided it would be easier to get married earlier than spend money going out. I remember with astonishment that we got married after only a very few months to save money having to go out.

We didn't have children straightaway. Neither of our parents owned their own home and it was really important for us to have the stability of our own home because we were both in a position of having to care for our parents. By this stage my Dad had had both legs amputated so that my parents really didn't leave their home except when I took them out. I used to have Thursdays off and we would do the shopping and all those things on Thursday. Also, within about six months of us getting married my husband's father had a stroke and was in hospital and then convalescent homes, so essentially my wage went to paying for the physio and the speech therapist each week. It all meant that for us to get our own home was really important because if these things happened to us we would have our own place and our kids wouldn't be in the position that we were in. We didn't mind, we probably thought we were fairly noble, doing all of this, and we were young enough, but it was a difficult situation that we didn't want our own kids to have.

We had an agreement that we were going to have eight kids. It was at least going to be a large family because I was an only child. Bob had three siblings but they were spaced out and his older sister was twenty years older than him. We had this ideal family concept which was a house full of kids fairly close together where we all did wonderful things together. I am sure that is what Bob tried valiantly to create with the kids that we did have because he continually tried to do the best thing for all of us which mostly ended up being awful things like putting us all in the car on the weekend and taking us on long drives to nowhere so we could be 'a family' together.

After a year or so Bob decided that it would be a good move for him to go into his own business. That meant that I would be working longer than originally envisaged, but with his father and all the other things, we decided I would do that. So he went into partnership in a service station.

I supported him in that, but I still had in my head the idea that we had an agreement that as soon as we got into our own house, as soon as we had the four walls, even if we ate off packing crates, we would start a family. But it kept getting put off and off and off and it was actually six years after we got married that we had our first baby. For me that was a real letdown even though I could see the logic of us doing it the way we had done it. It seemed to be the right thing to do but there was no real opportunity to talk about it happening. The other thing was that my husband's partner had just gone through a really messy divorce and all the worst attitudes to women which came out of that divorce came home to us, so that by the time we had kids there were real problems about our partnership of marriage. It was no longer a partnership, 'women were dirt' and 'would get you as much as they could'. I transferred most of my affection to the kids as they came. I had Christopher in 1972 and a little girl, Robin, in 1973.

Then Bob decided he didn't want any more kids. I was desperate for at least a third. Contraception was left up to me, which is just so crazy when you look back. There were quite valid contra-indications to the pill and I hated the idea of an IUD and although I was using cream or something, it failed and we had darling Carolyn which was a huge issue because one of my friends told Bob that I had done it on purpose. He loved her when it was a fait accompli but at the time he was very, very angry.

There were just continual things that separated him and me and I nursed all these resentments. We didn't ever talk through anything, we'd just argue.

I loved being a mother, especially of little children. I love being a mother now of older children but, at that time, being a mother was the first thing I had felt successful at.

We moved into Bob's parents' house. It had been decided much earlier that the house was to be left to us to make up for the assistance we had given over the years and then it turned out that rates hadn't been paid for ten years. There would be no house if we waited too long so, again, we did the sensible thing and bought the house. Along with that deal came Mother-in-law, who lived with us for fifteen years or longer. That meant that when I had my kids, when I came home with them – and mothering and breast-feeding was the only thing I had ever felt successful at – I had a mother-in-law sitting opposite me all the time. She just sat there and watched and told me what I did wrong.

I threw myself into the Nursing Mothers' Association. I still didn't have a sense of the way society is structured or how things hang together. Each incident was an incident and then you had another incident and there was almost no connection between one day and the next, there was no sense of building knowledge or building your life. I threw myself into the Nursing Mothers' Association because it was something I was passionate about, I could do it with the kids, and it would take me away from all of this.

They needed a group leader, someone to organise the local area, because the current one was moving, so I said I wouldn't mind doing that. I never felt competent to do anything so it was very much, if you don't mind too much I'll try and do it. I started doing the training and leading the group, and it was fantastic. Usually the training lasted for about eighteen months, but I kept going for four years.

There were some difficulties with the local hospital and the advice they were giving so I decided the way around this was to invite the key person at the hospital to come and talk to the mothers, to get her into our environment so that at least she had to hear what the mothers had to say. This worked so well that it was seen as a great breakthrough and I suddenly became the community educator for the state. These kinds of things have continually astonished me through Nursing Mothers because it seems to me that I just look at a situation, look for a solution and do it and suddenly I find it is some new innovative thing that becomes the model for the country.

That essentially was what Nursing Mothers was for me. I worked locally, then I went on to state involvement and was on a number of community education and public relations exercises with schools and the hospitals and so forth. I was deputy state president and then I stood for the national board of directors and got elected as honorary secretary the first year. I was vice president for two years and I was on the board for nine years. During that time I organised dozens of conferences and was part of the group that organised the first ever international conference on breast-feeding. That pulled in community groups from all around the world, which had never been done before. I established National Mothering Week which is still an annual event, the week before Mothers' Day, and Breast-feeding Awareness Month every October. I know I gave a lot to Nursing Mothers, but I got such a lot out of it. It was an open door. Whatever you wanted to do, if you could convince the people that it was a good thing, you could do it. It was wonderful in that way.

It was all voluntary and because it was national the phone bills were astronomical. There would be thousand-dollar phone bills. To a large degree I paid to do the work.

My husband allowed it. Which is a word I would apply to a lot of the other women. They were 'allowed' to come to meetings at nights. 'My husband doesn't mind if I come out at night.' It wasn't that we had a right, which is what I hear women say at meetings now, those same meetings. There is no question about being 'allowed' most of the time now.

Bob used to not like me going out at night so I would try and arrange meetings for the daytime as far as I could. At night he would sit at the other end of a very big room watching television with his back to me and I would sit at the table with piles of paperwork all around me, and this was 'family'. We never spoke unless we absolutely had to and the meal was got over as quickly as possible. The kids would be off to bed or playing in their own rooms or something. As long as I was in the same room it seemed to be somehow called normal family.

In 1979 my mother died, after my father had died five years earlier, and for me that was a huge shock. A lot of things happened that year that were really profound. I went to pick her up on the Thursday to go shopping and she was dead in bed. There was nobody who was mine any more. People kept telling me, you've got your own lovely little family, you've got a husband that loves you, and you've got these children. But I can remember standing at her graveside — it was a very windy day, and there was a tree blowing in the wind — and I thought, I'm like the trunk of that tree, and the kids are the branches but if you blow on me I'll fall over, there are no roots. I am sure I was in shock for a long time. That was the year I started National Mothering Week. For a lot of that year I hardly needed any sleep. I would work right through the night and into the next day. I didn't need much to eat or drink either, I was quite manic. I couldn't deal with the stuff from Mum's house. I had it all just packed as it was and put into storage.

We did rather well in the 'upwardly mobile stakes' through the 1970s and into the early 1980s. Bob had moved out of the garage and gone to work for a local car dealer and he had risen from car salesman through the management ranks so that he was actually general manager around that time. We sold the house at Asquith and bought a house at Castle Hill.

To me, this was the house that we bought with the proceeds from the house that Mum had been in, which we had financed but she had made the payments on. This house was incredibly symbolic of all the things that we had been striving for through the years. It was the biggest house in the street, on the highest block. It had five bedrooms and three bathrooms and a big area for Mother-in-law to be in, which was more separate than anything we had previously. Everything was brand-new. Bob wanted brand-new furniture and I was surrounded with Mum's furniture. Some of it I had to put into cupboards to hide, so I could keep it, because he wanted laminated chipboard. So, although the house was a symbol of success and status, it was also a symbol of my mother's death. We were only able to have it because I didn't have her any more. I enjoyed the house but it was an incredibly sad place. I used one of the bedrooms as my study and from it you could see all the kids in the cul-de-sac going from one house to another. I would sit there and watch them and they would come over to my place and it was my turn to be Mum to them all for a while. It could have been a lovely environment, but it wasn't.

I found there were an awful lot of other unhappy women as well. I recall one incident at Christmas time. I had a call as a Nursing Mothers' breast-feeding counsellor from a young Asian-sounding woman who had a new baby at home and she asked if I could come and visit because we couldn't communicate easily enough over the phone to solve the problem. I went out to her house, and it was a glamorous place with columns in front, a fountain and a circular driveway, all those things, but when I went through the front door — there was no inside to the house, there was no stairway to the second storey, they were sleeping on a mattress on the floor in the hallway. I thought, this is so symbolic of bloody Castle Hill — it's all facade.

One of the things I did there was go to the community health centre and ask if they had self-esteem courses. I had done some on the north side and I thought I could really do with a refresher. There were a lot of others around that I had spoken to who had said they would be really interested in it too. I left my name and a couple of weeks later they asked if I would be interested in running them. So I ended up becoming a community educator with the local health service running self-esteem courses and that was wonderful. There was probably a fifty-per-cent divorce rate at the end of each course and it was mostly because women didn't come until they were just so, so distraught that they had to make a commitment.

I had to negotiate with Bob to get the job. It was just four hours once a week, for eight weeks, three times a year, so it wasn't a major job but Bob saw it as a threat to his being the breadwinner. The argument he used was that it was going to mess up his tax and that stopped me for probably three or four months until I found somebody who could explain what this really meant. Until recently, when the dependent spouse rebate has been got rid of, bundled up into the childcare allowance and so on, that has been a huge political tool within households, just as it was for me. I was bamboozled by that for quite a time.

When I finally took the job, I can remember that the tension was really bad. By that stage we were very unhappy at home, we were all frustrated. I was absent most of the time, at least in my head, if not a lot of the time in practice. One of the measures of housewifeliness for Bob was that when he came home the house was neat and tidy and there was food on the table and he used to expect it at six o'clock every afternoon. From five to six o'clock every day that house was just turmoil and chaos. The three kids and I tore around the house to get everything in order before Dad came home so he wouldn't be angry when he got home, and there was always something wrong. The tension was just dreadful.

Then I got pregnant again and it was quite a shock. It was by no means planned and I decided that there was no way I could bring a baby into those circumstances. I decided we had to fix it or we had to end it so I marched us all off to family therapy. The kids would never go to therapy again for anything after those awful family therapy sessions. They didn't work so we separated in the same house for a year. First of all I said that Bob's mother had to go. We had had arguments about his mother for years and she was always so sick that you couldn't put her anywhere else. However, when it came to the crunch, well over ten years after she had come to live with us, Bob got a flat for her and she actually lived in the flat for five or six years after that. When she went, Bob had the top half of the house and I had the bottom half. We lived like that for about a year and then I needed him to go, I was nearly going mad. He moved out and we sold the house.

Almost as soon as I made the decision that the marriage was finished and I told Bob that, I had a miscarriage. I haemorrhaged really badly and I had one of those out-of-body experiences. Bob, trying to do the right thing again, took the kids to a friend up on the Central Coast so, at the moment when I needed to hold my children, nobody was there. He always did try and do the right thing and it always seemed to me to be most inappropriate. I don't know what to make of that. I make different things at different times.

We moved to Mount Colah, just me and the kids, into a house that had been eaten out by white ants. We had virtually nothing but there was enough money to replace the white-ant-eaten bit, although not to paint it. Bob was good with the maintenance for the kids, that was there regularly, but it was very difficult to get anything extra and it really was never enough. There were quite a few times when there wasn't money for the kids to go on excursions and to have the proper clothing. They got quite adept at going to the right people at school and whispering that they needed some help.

We were all incredibly traumatised and had used violence for so long to deal with problems that it took a long time to get over that. As far as my marriage was concerned, I had blocked a lot of it out. It was emotionally violent always but I can remember telling a friend about a time when I was pinned against a wall and choked and she said, 'But this happened to you last month too.' I couldn't remember it happening last month because I always, like all good women, took responsibility for making the relationship work. I kept trying to put the bad stuff behind and make tomorrow okay. But over a period of time I started to see that of course there was some physical violence there. Particularly with the kids. It seemed that we always needed to know who was responsible for any little thing so the kids were always set up in opposition to each other, they hated each other, they couldn't trust each other, they had no bonds. We took all of that stuff with us to Mount Colah. I declared the place a non-violent house so that when different ones of us did go off the deep end, everybody else had permission to stop it happening. There was a lot of trauma and a lot of healing to do.

In 1988 I got a call from Margaret Reynolds, who was Women's Minister in the federal government at the time, inviting me to represent Nursing Mothers on the National Women's Consultative Council which I thought was absolutely wonderful and said yes to. Then I sat down and thought, my God, she said representing the women of Australia and I'm not sure I know very much about women at all, except for the women I've worked with. So I rang the Women's Electoral Lobby and said, 'Please help, I know about babies and boobs, but who else can I talk to?' They put me in touch with Eva Cox and I went to see her and we had this incredible three hours where I took notes and she just kept talking and that was the beginning of a wonderful friendship and mentorship. Eva just walked me into feminist circles.

Round about that time, when Paul Keating was Treasurer, he announced that there were going to be some tax cuts for high-income people. When I came back from the meeting Eva said, 'You know, this means that most women are going to miss out on these tax cuts; this is really, really important, this is something that women should do something about.' So we rallied WEL nationally and I talked to the National Women's Consultative Council and after various meetings it was decided that there would be a joint NWCC and WEL women's tax summit, like the tax summit when Hawke first came in. Then the Council asked me, with all my vast conference organising experience, to organise it in a paid capacity. The day they asked me Eva was in Melbourne, and I can remember vividly ringing her up, getting her out of the conference and saying, 'They have asked me to organise this conference,' which was going to be a bringing-together of all the major organisations, two or three hundred women, in Parliament House in Canberra. She said, 'Terrific, you can do that,' and I said, 'Yes, but they want to pay me.' She said, 'For heaven's sake, take it!' I still haven't received the whole amount because I just found it so hard to accept money for doing stuff that I had done for nothing for so long. It's crazy, isn't it?

As for this time of my life, now, I just love it. I have done a bit of uni, I have done a few other things, I can see the spread of things. I know that structure is really important for me now. If I can plot where things are, I know exactly what to do and that's being this age. I also think that because I have experienced all that I have, all the disjointedness and the sadness and the ups and the downs, I have an optimism about being able to do things that a lot of other women my age don't seem to have. A lot of what I experienced in the voluntary field taught me that if you don't know the background of things you often just do them, whereas if you know what the obstacles are you would never start. It does create a few problems because for me, quite often, achieving a goal is so clear and I don't explain too well because it's so clear.

The other thing is that what the neighbours might think doesn't matter too much any more. Bugger that! Also, I go to work now. When I started work in the Public Service two years ago Eva took me out and bought me all this wonderful whizzbang gear that public servants wear, shoulder pads, the lot. Look at me now, flat shoes, slacks and a jacket, because I am really happy to be who I am and I just stand on who I am. I love that.

I have also got a house of my own now and that's come with the fifties. What's bad? I think I am just revelling in it!

I have to say my health's gone down the tube. I've developed late onset diabetes and my eyesight isn't wonderful and I know I can't lift the physical weights that I used to and things like that. But I have also got a wee bit more money so I hire a man to do that. If I am really feeling sick then yes, I'll think, this is to do with age and I know that this type of diabetes is to do with age but it's not debilitating. In fact, it is a bit of a trigger to be healthy because I am eating properly, exercising and I have stopped smoking so these things can be positive. I choose for them to be positive.

As far as menopause is concerned, I didn't have a period after I had the miscarriage. Essentially, I carked it for a couple of minutes and while they were waiting for the doctor to arrive they pumped blood into me, they actually got blood out of the fridge and put it in three different places and squeezed it in and it really mucked up the whole thermostat system of my body for two or three years afterwards. I'd get hot or cold at different times and I never had a period again. So for menopause as such, I had a few hot sweats but it wasn't anything.

In general, I think menopause is something like post-natal depression. We live such crazy lives that of course we react to that craziness in some ways that look crazy. If we had more supports around us and more women around us doing the same sort of thing as some other societies do, where they can go off to their women's house and deal with these things together, we may react to it differently. I think that there are whole industries around these parts of women's reproductive lives that have to beat it all up in order to justify their own existence. When you are feeling low, it's really easy to intensify that. As an example of the other side of the coin, Betty Friedan says that she missed menopause, she was too busy, she thinks she had a hot flush one day. I know that there are women who have real problems. There is a real hormonal thing happening but there's also all the other stuff. It's very hard to tell the difference.

I am really looking forward to getting older. One thing I have had a lot to do with is the Older Women's Network and I can see what's there in the future. I felt really good when I turned forty. I was in Nursing Mothers then and I felt as if it was a real rite of passage from doing the learning, being the learner, to being the wiser person who has the experience. You've achieved a milestone. That's really what I am thinking mostly about in terms of turning fifty and moving onwards from there. There are just such wonderful role models. If I look at some of the women I really admire like Edna Ryan [prominent feminist and author, aged ninety], age hasn't stopped them doing what they want to do, so what's the problem?

My job at the Office on Ageing is mostly about the issue of the image of ageing and media images in particular. The media generally doesn't bother about older people. Older people really don't exist in the media or, if they do, it's the negative stereotype. If older people don't see themselves reflected in the mainstream of life through the papers or on television or whatever, or if they only see themselves when they are victims of something or when they are a burden on society, it really affects their capacity to live whole lives so my job is to try and do something about media portrayal. The state government has put in place age discrimination legislation both for retirement – you can't make people retire at a certain age any more – and employment generally, and all the other things that are covered by the anti-discrimination legislation, but underlying that are people's attitudes. You might change their behaviour with the legislation but it is the attitudes that I have to deal with. We have done things like setting up the Seniors' Media Network, getting together through a whole series of strategies, media people and older people, getting them into dialogue with each other. The government has been the vehicle to create the opportunities for that to happen. We have now got a Council that is headed by Ita Buttrose which is doing it in an ongoing way. That is one strand. Another strand is the Premier's Forum on Ageing which is an opportunity for older people to come in and actually have a say. Today we had a workshop for the workshop leaders to get them to make sure everybody has a chance to have a say and that they finish up with outcomes that we can actually action by government. We must show the way, create the plan, and then older people themselves can create their own way forward. Recently we had an EPAC [Economic Planning and Advisory Committee] report on Australia's ageing population. The report itself is actually quite even-handed — it talks about the negatives and the positives — but what hit the general public through the media was that we are in a real pickle because of all of these older people. That is not necessarily the situation and if the plans are made on that perception they are going to be totally inappropriate plans. A lot of older people would love to be in the paid workforce and paying taxes or underpinning the paid workforce by providing all the voluntary labour that is around. There are lots of issues so creating things like the Premier's Forum where the plans or how policy can be made come from the older people themselves and their perspective as well as all the other sectors is important. Things like Seniors' Week used to be almost bread and circuses and now the grants program is targeted at community organisations who will not only put on a dinner but will also create some event which actually acknowledges that 'use it or lose it' is true. Just doling out stuff isn't terribly helpful for older people. We should provide something where they can actually interact with each other and interact with younger generations, build bridges across the generations. So all the activities are much more towards bringing older people — the enclave of 'the elderly' — back into a sense of the whole community and not being off there beyond the pale. Because they are not that.

I am optimistic about the future because futures are made by creating the dream that you want it to be and working at getting it there. If you are not going to be optimistic about it then it is not going to happen. There are a whole lot of things that I think need to happen and really fundamental things that are beginning to happen globally, for example, looking at what kind of global environment we can sustain and which provides us with the kind of life that we would value. How do we value things in the world? If we only value money transactions and things that the International Monetary Fund and the World Bank and the System of National Accounts count, then it can't work because all of that is based on a formula that was good after World War II, in 1945. It doesn't equate with now. Some of those real fundamentals have to be changed and they are beginning to change. Even the fact that people are now identifying that there is a problem is a huge leap from five years ago. So some of those really fundamental things will change and I think feminism itself is looking less at critiquing patriarchy, although that will continue, and more at creating a feminist future. The 1980s are a real example of when you haven't got clear in your own mind what you want, you just lurch from one bad scenario to another within a very limited framework. Creating our own futures will bring a future.

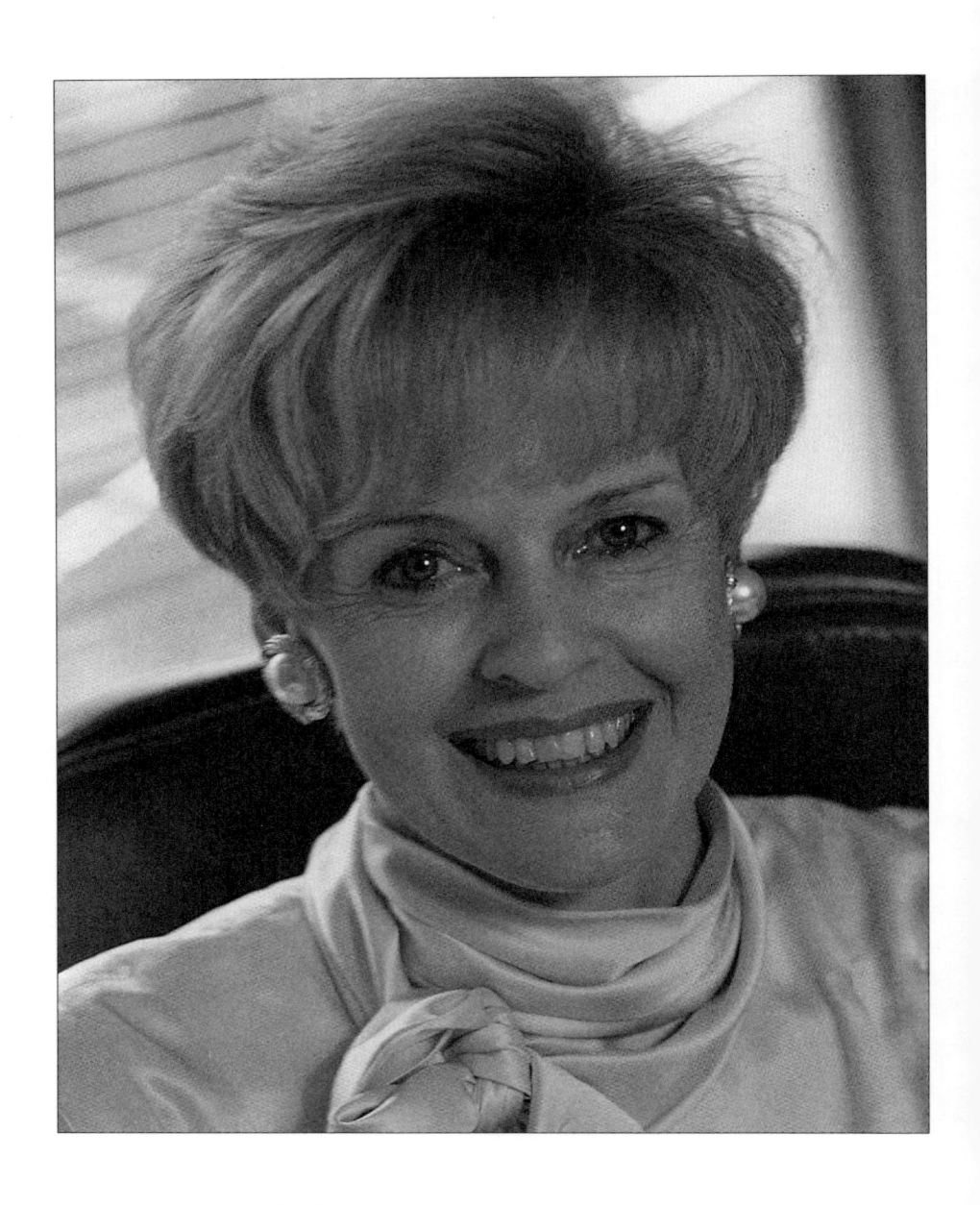

*We have seen a social revolution in our lifetime,
in every aspect of Australian society. We need to celebrate that and to
remember how far we have come.*

❖ ❖ ❖

Quentin Bryce

My meeting with Quentin Bryce took place on a bitterly cold winter's morning when I went to her National Childcare Accreditation Council office in Sydney's CBD. As we greeted one another, she grasped both my hands and rubbed them between her own — 'Ooh, you're cold!' — a motherly gesture which clearly came from a lifetime of rearing five children. It was completely unselfconscious and I found myself thinking how many dimensions successful women often have. It is difficult to imagine being greeted by a male chief executive in such a way. Jibes about possible sexual harassment charges aside, such human concern is rarely part of the top management male ethos.

On the face of it at least, Quentin is a woman who has it all. A successful marriage, a large and loving family and a fulfilling career. She is also strikingly beautiful. Tall and slim, with fashionably short blonde-tipped hair and wearing on this day, a dusty-pink silk blouse under a charcoal-grey pantsuit with high-heeled black boots, she was the epitome of elegance. Her calm manner makes it hard to imagine that she ever gets fazed by anything. And yet she says she 'beats herself up under the shower' for mistakes she makes. She maintains that 'men handle the ups and downs of life much better: they say, "that was a cock up," and get on with the next thing', an ability she envies.

Quentin seems always to have had a very clear sense of where she is going. In an era when it was still rare for a woman to go to university and arts was considered the only suitable area of study for those who did manage to overcome prevailing social attitudes and prejudices, Quentin did law. She was one of the first women in Queensland to graduate in that discipline and be admitted to the Bar. Then she saw no reason why she should not combine marriage and motherhood with her chosen career, and for some fifteen years was a lecturer in law at Queensland University Law School, having been the first woman appointed to the staff of that faculty. At the same time as all this she reared not just one or two, but five children.

It is not surprising that she became acutely aware of the difficulties facing women in her position. What is amazing, given the obviously huge demands on her time and attention in combining work and increasing family responsibilities, is that she did something about it and joined others in her community in voluntary activity to establish services and programs for children and their families.

That involvement with women and children continued to evolve at a more formal level and has been the linchpin of her entire professional life. Quentin was the first national president of the Association for the Welfare of Children in Hospital. She has worked in the areas of juvenile justice, mandatory reporting of child abuse, legal representation of children and adoption law reform. In 1979 she was awarded a scholarship by the US State Department to study children's programs in the United States and she has lectured and written widely in these areas, particularly in the field of child safety legislation.

In 1988 Quentin was a member of Australia's delegation to the United Nations Commission for Human Rights in Geneva for its debate on the Rights of the Child. In the same year, she was made an Officer of the Order of Australia for her services to children.

In 1984 Quentin established the Queensland Women's Information Service, as part of the Department of the Prime Minister and Cabinet and in 1987 she was appointed director of the Human Rights and Equal Opportunity Commission in Queensland. In 1988 she sprang to national prominence when she became federal Sex Discrimination Commissioner.

In her spare time Quentin has been a member, and ultimately convenor, of the National Women's Advisory Council. Her work for the Council included convening Queensland conferences to mark the mid decade for women, a national conference for mothers of disabled children, and consultations with Aboriginal women.

From 1982 to 1986 Quentin was women's representative to the National Committee on Discrimination in Employment and Occupation. In 1983 she was appointed Commonwealth representative on the board of the Australian Children's Television Foundation.

At an international level, Quentin has been delegate to numerous conferences concerning women and children including in 1993 the Lawyers Committee for Civil Rights Conference in Johannesburg, South Africa.

Currently, Quentin is a director of the Mindcare Mental Health Foundation, the Family Planning Council of Queensland and the Schizophrenia Foundation of Australia. She is a member of the International Women's Rights Action Watch, the Centre of Australian Public Sector Management Advisory Committee Queensland, the Visiting Committee of Griffith Law School, the National Institute for Law, Ethics and Public Affairs Advisory Board at Queensland's Griffith University, and the Australian Institute of Women's Research and Policy.

But Quentin's main role, now, is as chief executive and chairperson of the National Childcare Accreditation Council, an organisation established to ensure quality childcare standards, over and above basic licensing requirements. The job represents the full turn of the wheel in Quentin's life. Thirty years after she began such activity at a grassroots community level, she is now working for a government instrumentality seeking to guarantee that children receive the best care possible outside their family environment. For Quentin, good quality childcare is a human rights matter. She points out that the issue is no longer about children being minded for a few hours a day: some children are in long day care for almost as many hours as they spend in their primary and secondary schooling. 'That is what throws the quality of it into such sharp focus. If they are going to be there, we must make it the very best experience possible.'

It is apparent even now that Quentin has an astonishing range of interests and activities. A week or so after our meeting she was due to participate in a book fair in Melbourne, chairing a session on the future of the information industry vis à vis computers. Expressing some misgivings about the undertaking since she was, by her own admission, a 'computer ignoramus', she was nevertheless undeterred. She said that she thought she would probably inject some humour into the proceedings by using a laptop as a support for painting her nails!

I was surprised during our meeting when Quentin said that she had not really 'got going' until her mid-forties, a mere seven or eight years ago. She seems to have been upfront on the national stage for much longer than that. I recall hearing her speak at a conference some fifteen years ago (on the law and computers!). Perhaps it depends on one's definition of 'getting going'.

Quentin makes it clear that family has always come first for her. And yet it has clearly not been, as it was for so many women of her generation, at the expense of having a life of her own.

Essentially, Quentin now lives in Sydney at the same time as maintaining her family home in Brisbane where her graphic designer husband, Michael Bryce, remains. She intends to return there at some time in the reasonably foreseeable future to tend her beloved garden (another interest!) and give her daughter support, in particular working part-time while she minds her (as yet unborn) grandchildren so that her daughter, in her turn, can combine a fulfilling career and intellectual achievement with having a family.

✢ ✢ ✢

The decades have been broken up in my life in a fairly convenient sort of way. The 1950s for me was my schooling and then in 1960 I went to Queensland University where I did an arts/law degree. I was called to the Bar in 1965, a few days after I had graduated in law, and those were very important experiences in terms of later influences and opportunities in my life.

I was married in 1964, when I was a student, at the end of my fifth year at university. I finished off university and by that time, I was expecting my first child. I went to live in Europe with my husband and had a couple of years there. When I came back to Australia, I brought with me another child, my first daughter, who was born in England. I came back to Brisbane and started working in a way in which very many women of my generation did, on a part-time basis. I started tutoring in law at Queensland University, and I also enrolled for a higher degree. I was feeling very much that it was time I got on with my career and all the things that I wanted to do. I had always assumed that I would be able to do everything — that I would be able to have a fulfilling career and that I would be able to combine that with family responsibilities. When I came back to Australia I was conscious of the need to get on with things, that while my husband had been having a significant professional and postgraduate experience, I had been full-time mothering, which I enjoyed very much, but I wanted to do something besides that. So I went to the university to enrol in a higher degree. I had always been a pretty successful student and had done well academically and that was the first thing that came to mind.

I tutored part-time. I used to go for a couple of hours, two days a week, and that meant getting into the world of childcare and here I am, back in it, thirty years later. Now in my fifties there are a lot of things that I have done in the past that tie in with what I am doing now. My life seems to have been a series of circles, intersecting circles.

Also, like a lot of other women of my generation, I moved from part-time work into full-time work because of the extraordinary forms of discrimination and disadvantages of part-time work. I was working at a casual rate — I think it was three dollars an hour — tutoring in the Law School. It was a bit of a shock to the Law School because they hadn't had a woman on the staff and especially not one who was a mother and was pregnant and talked about breast-feeding and being pregnant. Even the presence of a person like that in that environment was a shock, and in many ways it was a pretty isolating experience for me. I remember going to see the head of the department to complain about my remuneration and he just said, 'Look, there's nothing I can do about it.' What I had discovered was that I was being paid this extraordinarily small amount of money and people who were on a full-time basis, with fewer student–teacher contact hours, and who had a lesser workload, were earning much more and had access to things like superannuation. Of course this was all in the days before any semblance of equal pay and not long after the marriage bar had been lifted. I stayed in academic life, moving very slowly, extremely slowly, at snail's pace up the academic ladder. There were all the challenges and difficulties and frustrations about work and family life that I didn't notice much at the time. I was so busy, and running so fast, because I had five children under seven, and I moved into some of the terrible superwoman tag stuff from which I have always been at pains to distance myself, and it was all pretty awful. But it was also a time when I learned a lot of very important lessons about myself and the world and the world of work. Particularly with respect to my health, because at one stage I became quite ill when I was trying to do too much, going home breast-feeding through the day, and looking after the family. Certainly I had help, but it was minimal, not enough, and my husband had enormous pressures establishing a small professional practice. I was running a pretty busy social life as well, with dinner parties and everything. My God, the dinner parties we used to have in the 1970s! I became quite ill, and I remember sitting in a tutorial one day actually wearing my old rabbity fur coat from England shivering, with burning cheeks, trying to give a tutorial. Since then I don't think I have ever had a day that I've been sick. It really taught me about looking after my health and what I eat, pacing myself, and it's something I'm now evangelical about with young women, particularly mothers, who I see trying to do too much.

I became involved in an enormous range of community work while I was at university. That was the up side of being an academic and not getting much job satisfaction there. All these things happened in a fairly natural way, for example, being involved in establishing children's services of all kinds, the things I needed for my family, because they weren't around. That was very important for me too because I made friends then with the women who are still my closest, lifelong friends. I haven't seen them much over the last few years because their lives have always been very different from mine but I am seeing them again now. I was the only 'working mother', as we were called, in the group at that time, but they were extraordinarily supportive to me. They used to say things to me like, we're a bit fed up with your working mother's guilt. All this was at a time when there was a very clear message from society that working mothers were greedy, aberrant, wicked, taking jobs away from boys and, very importantly, not good mothers. It's always the important thing for a mother, to be considered to be a good enough mother. There was all the talk of latch-key kids, that the children of working mothers would be failures and delinquents, and those things are very much on my mind now because of my present job, visiting long-day-care centres. It gives me the opportunity to pause and reflect on those times and how significant they were in our lives, in our family's lives and the remarkable friendships that came out of those times. Also, the support from women in the long-day-care centres. I look back on how supportive they were to me, how then they tended to be older women and we were younger mothers and they nurtured the mothers as much as they nurtured the children.

I was invited to get involved in a lot of community issues because I was a lawyer and there weren't many around like me who were interested and committed to children's issues and family issues. I just went on doing more and more work in the voluntary sector, in child advocacy and children-in-hospital work and things that came along that I was interested in, that were important to me and where I was able to make a contribution. I learned an enormous amount and they were my first experiences of political life in a very hostile climate in Queensland where everything about change was opposed.

I went on with academic work until the early 1980s. I left the university in about 1982 or 1983 when I was appointed to a very interesting job in Queensland by the Office of the Status of Women which was part of the Department of the Prime Minister and Cabinet in Canberra. When the federal Labor government came in, the Hawke government, they decided to set up a Women's Information Service in Queensland because there were no programs and policies for Queensland women. The most significant of those federal initiatives was what was then the Sex Discrimination Bill. So I had a long relationship with that reform before it actually went into legislation. I was there at the Women's Information Service for a number of years and that was a wonderful time, it was exhilarating. Then I had about a year running the Human Rights and Equal Opportunity Commission office in Queensland, where I was administering the Sex Discrimination Act, the Race Discrimination Act and other human rights instruments. Then, at the beginning of 1988, I was appointed federal Sex Discrimination Commissioner.

That was a very challenging job. It is now the tenth anniversary of the Act and it is extraordinary to look back and think about its very controversial introduction and to see, now, the way it is well settled into the mainstream of Australian society. What strikes me is how in ten years you can really bring about changes in attitudes and behaviour and have successful educative programs. I think it is remarkable what the Act has achieved. Having responsibility for it for five years was a very exciting challenge but it was also very hard work, really tough going.

As the cliché goes, 'we have come a long way'. Just looking back from when I started work, when I graduated, there have been extraordinary changes in terms of equality. People didn't even talk about it much when I was at university, there were references to suffragettes and that was about it. We've seen a social revolution in our lifetime, in every aspect of Australian society. I think we need to celebrate that and to remember how far we have come. It's tough times in many ways now and we need to celebrate those achievements, to be aware of them, to have in our minds all the good news, the positive things, because although there has been a social revolution and remarkable change, we still are a long way from equality. I think perhaps that the last phase is the hardest. Getting to eighty per cent of equal pay, for example, moving from fifty to eighty per cent, that has been tough and it has taken a long time. I think those last steps are going to be very hard ones because there is this assumption that because it has changed so much, women have made it, that they do have equality. I hear these undertones of, what are you lot whingeing about? and, well, we've fixed up that problem! and, it's a joke to talk about women's rights as minority rights, because there are now women in jobs where they weren't even five or ten years ago — judges and cabinet ministers, heads of unions, women priests in one church — and so that's it, we've done it all. Then there's another school of thought who think that now it will just all happen, we've come so far it will all just eventually evolve. I don't take anything for granted at all. I think that we are going to need an enormous amount of energy just to keep on the march until we do have true equality and equal status and equal opportunities.

I don't agree that young women are opting out, though. Just this morning in the newspaper there is a photograph of four young girls — they're about thirteen or so, with smiling fresh faces — saying they're going to take over the world and it's time that men stayed at home and sacrificed their careers. They are the sort of gutsy, confident girls around now. There was a program too on *Four Corners* [ABC television] about now girls are doing so well at school we have got to have all these special programs for boys. Just watching the girls in that program, at the school, the way they were so articulate, I have enormous confidence that some of them will carry on. It has only ever been some women, a few women, who have been active participants in the women's movement. There are certainly four in the *Sydney Morning Herald* and these girls today are just so delightfully confident and stand up for themselves and know that they do have rights, and know how to exercise them. I hear people sitting around despairing of young women who don't want to be called feminists and you hear lines like, they don't understand how hard it's been for us, and, they don't know that when they go out there they'll be discriminated against. I don't think that they have to be coming to our women's meetings. Why would young women want to come to middle-aged women's meetings? They never did. The idea of going to my mother's meetings would have totally bored me to sobs. In my family I have two daughters who describe themselves as feminists, their friends talk about feminist issues and all the things that we would have talked about in relation to equality, and they complain about things and plan things and want to be involved, but they certainly don't want to do it with us. And they'll do it differently. But I don't worry that they don't know their history, they don't understand it was so hard and they take things for granted. I think it's good that they take things for granted and that they go out in the world confident and articulate. I don't want to be saying to them, 'Oooh, it'll be tough on you out there, you'll be discriminated against.' I think they should go out there expecting everything will be good and holding their heads up and demanding their rights and saying, this isn't good enough! Confidence is such an important thing because all through our lifetime we have talked about girls' lack of self-esteem and our own doubts and so I think it is a wonderful thing that has happened.

I do think that there is a glass ceiling. I think it's a very perceptive term because I see a lot of women who have hit that glass ceiling. It is tied up with a whole lot of things like, well, women have made it now, and, we've done enough for them, and some discriminatory attitudes and some prejudice from men who feel very uncomfortable with women in senior positions. There is still a lot of that around. Women are not welcomed and accepted and recognised in a lot of workplaces and I detect quite a bit of, well, we've got these women in senior positions now and we'll just go back to our old boys' club practices, we don't really want them in there with us, because they do feel uncomfortable with them. Certainly that will change too but I know men of my age group, my peers, there are a lot of them who feel uncomfortable, they cannot relate to women as colleagues and as friends, they still have those old stereotypical attitudes and prejudices that they grew up with and they can't throw them off.

Turning fifty happened to me at an interesting time because it represented a time of transition, of going from one phase of my life to another. At the time I turned fifty I was finishing up as Sex Discrimination Commissioner and it meant moving out of an area that I had had an intense commitment to for about ten years, much longer than being in the position itself. My elder daughter, my second child, was being married, I spent some time working in South Africa at an extraordinarily interesting time, and so for me it was all part of a transition from one phase in my life to another. But it wasn't something that caused me any angst. It didn't particularly upset me, I didn't have any great emotional response to it.

I suppose I see it as a sort of continuum in personal and professional growth and development. Certainly there is a sense of confidence and freedom, all those things, but that's something that has been gradually evolving for me prior to now. I think for me it probably started in my mid-forties, because my children were born when I was a young mother and when I was forty-five or so I took up my Sex Discrimination Commissioner's position. That meant very significant things for me in my life. It meant deciding to live in Sydney where I made my first attempt ever at living on my own. One of my younger sisters said to me in a rather perjorative way, 'Well, that's going to be a big challenge, you've moved from cocoon to cocoon,' — which was true. It was at fifty that I really moved into 'a room of my own', as it were. My husband and I both live between Sydney and Brisbane but I am in Sydney more and more with the jobs that I have had. They are all-encompassing and that is something I have really enjoyed very much — the opportunity to throw myself into my work. I don't admire my trait of workaholism but it is something I admire in others and I don't want to be a poor example to people who work with me.

The fifties have been terrific for me because it was the end of having to be endlessly making compromises about my career and work and family, a lot of those things that have been very hard. For me, the most important thing in my life has always been my family and it is marvellous that those responsibilities have changed, to have got them to adulthood, to be able to do other things. When I am away from them I don't think about them at all. I don't worry about them. They are all grown up now but when I came to Sydney in 1988 my youngest child was about fifteen. So for me it has been about being able to be myself, to put myself on the top of my agenda and that's been a wonderful thing to happen, and to be able to do what I like when I like. I still can't completely – obviously there are other people I have to think about all the time when I am making decisions about what I am going to do and how I am going to do it, but it is a real case of having a room of one's own. I have a little apartment here, I can go home when I like, I don't have to worry about anything when I get home. Just having time for reflection and controlling my own life has been an extraordinary change because I really did move from one cocoon to another. I was at boarding school and university and then I was married when I was twenty-one.

Getting older doesn't bother me at all. At present I feel stretched in a lot of ways and I find it very exciting having adult children. I find them really enjoyable and lots of fun, although not all the anxiety about them has disappeared. I agree with Margaret Drabble who once wrote a wonderful piece in *The New York Times* talking about motherhood being anxiety, and it is to me. I haven't cast all that off and in my mind they're not all safe and secure and on the road to full adulthood. But I enjoy their company very much and what they're doing and their successes and their trials. They are wonderful fun and I enjoy seeing an incredible camaraderie amongst them now. At the same time, like most fifty-year-old women, I have other family responsibilities too, all those other things that happen. There are a couple of people in my immediate family who are never out of my head at present. One, who is very ill, to whom I am very close and another one who is having a very bleak time, as well as two ageing mothers, a mother and a mother-in-law. Just even keeping in touch with them all is very time-consuming, but I enjoy it. Just a little while ago we had a wonderful family celebration for my aunt, my late father's last remaining sibling, who turned ninety. I love those occasions where the huge, rich, extended family that I belong to gets together and I made sure all my children came to it, so they could see all their cousins who are growing up in the next generation. Those things are very important to me and I have a sense of increasing responsibility there. I try to ring my mother regularly and have a long talk to her or sometimes it will be a very quick one. All that takes a lot of time. You never have enough time.

I find this job that I'm in at present very testing and very difficult, but it is something that is very important to me. One thing that has been a privilege in my working life is that I have always worked in things to which I have a deep personal commitment. The other side of that coin is that you do work yourself to death because you are very committed to the job and you never have the resources that you need so you do it yourself.

I don't think about getting old. I don't feel old. I've hardly got going. I didn't get going at all until I was in my forties. I think the other wonderful thing that we have seen in our lives is how different they are from our mothers and our grandmothers. Remember what they used to look like and what their lives were like when they were in their sixties. Darkened rooms and little lace collars and corsets and genteel manners and very constrained lives. Whereas the women in their forties and fifties that I know will continue into their sixties with great energy and enthusiasm and certainly increased confidence. I don't worry about a lot of the things that I used to. I feel a sense of liberation and I try not to flagellate myself for mistakes I make as much as I used to once. Some of the self-doubt goes.

I don't give a stuff about society's so-called attitude to older women. I think we will change it. We've changed so many other things and we're going to change that. With all the things that we have done in our lives, combining work and family, being involved in community things, having so much energy, getting to a stage where we can do more of what we really want to do, I think that will all keep going. I think that there are some really interesting times ahead and all the skills that we have acquired, under very difficult circumstances very often, those skills are going to stand us in great stead. For myself, I am looking forward to doing things I have never had time to do. Right down the track. I think, I'll wait until I am in my seventies to do that.

In some ways as you get older you have more energy. I am not as serious about my fitness as I should be, but I am conscious of it. I don't need as much sleep. I probably organise my time a bit better. I don't think of myself as old. I don't mean that in the context of denying my ageing at all. But I like it, I like this phase of my life, where my children are, and my work. That is not to say that everything is wonderful and there are not some things I wouldn't like to change, and some frustrations, and things that I want to change about myself, about the way that I live my life, but I love it, I don't feel any problems.

Physically ageing doesn't worry me at all. My mother-in-law, who is in her eighties, said to me recently that she feels exactly the same inside, she feels she is the same person, she doesn't see herself as any different at eighty-two from when she was my age. I think that's true. I just hope that I'm wiser and perhaps even a bit bolder.

I admire the bravery and the courage of women who say that if they had their time over again they wouldn't have children, because they help to break down the stereotypes that confine us and our choices. It is important for younger women to know that it's alright to say those things and to understand and to learn that you don't have to do things, you don't have to be confined to stereotypes and there are real choices. The women who say those things contribute to that.

For myself, I would like to have had one more child. I wanted to have a big family. I like them. I think that my children will all make a practical and true contribution to society. They are all intelligent and well-educated and they care about things and they are informed about all of the things that are important to me. They have got a very strong sense of values that have been part of the family they have been brought up in, and they have been a very rich source of happiness and enjoyment. That is not to say I haven't had extraordinary ups and downs and difficulties and all the things that parenthood is about. My children have had a very unusual father as well as an unusual mother. My husband has been very involved in their lives in a completely different way from his peers. When the children were little I certainly had most of the physical demands of parenthood in our family, but particularly from their teenage years he has got a lot of enjoyment out of it. He has been very involved in everything that they have done, in their sports, in their schools, all those things. In the last decade or so there has been a clear understanding in the family that it is my turn now and no feelings of guilt or underlying hostility about what I am doing and the fact that they are not really first any more. That has been a growing experience for all of them.

I think that a lot of children, in Australia, as they get older are over-mothered. I used to see it particularly at my boys' school, the women carrying their boys' bags and being up at the school being seen in roles of almost domestic servitude. I can't stand the way mothers — and it's certainly their choice and I respect it — but mothers are up there washing up the plates so the boys can go and play sport. That worries me, the continuation of these stereotype roles, the boys seeing their mothers doing the cleaning up, as it were. And the fathers — this is still happening everywhere in Australia — the fathers sit down on the river bank watching the rowing and the training, because they drive them, but the mothers are up there washing the dishes. I'd say this is the worst deployment of labour I have ever seen. Why don't these boys wash their own dishes! I think it is appalling in 1994 that that's still going on in so many places. What do they expect their wives to be like?

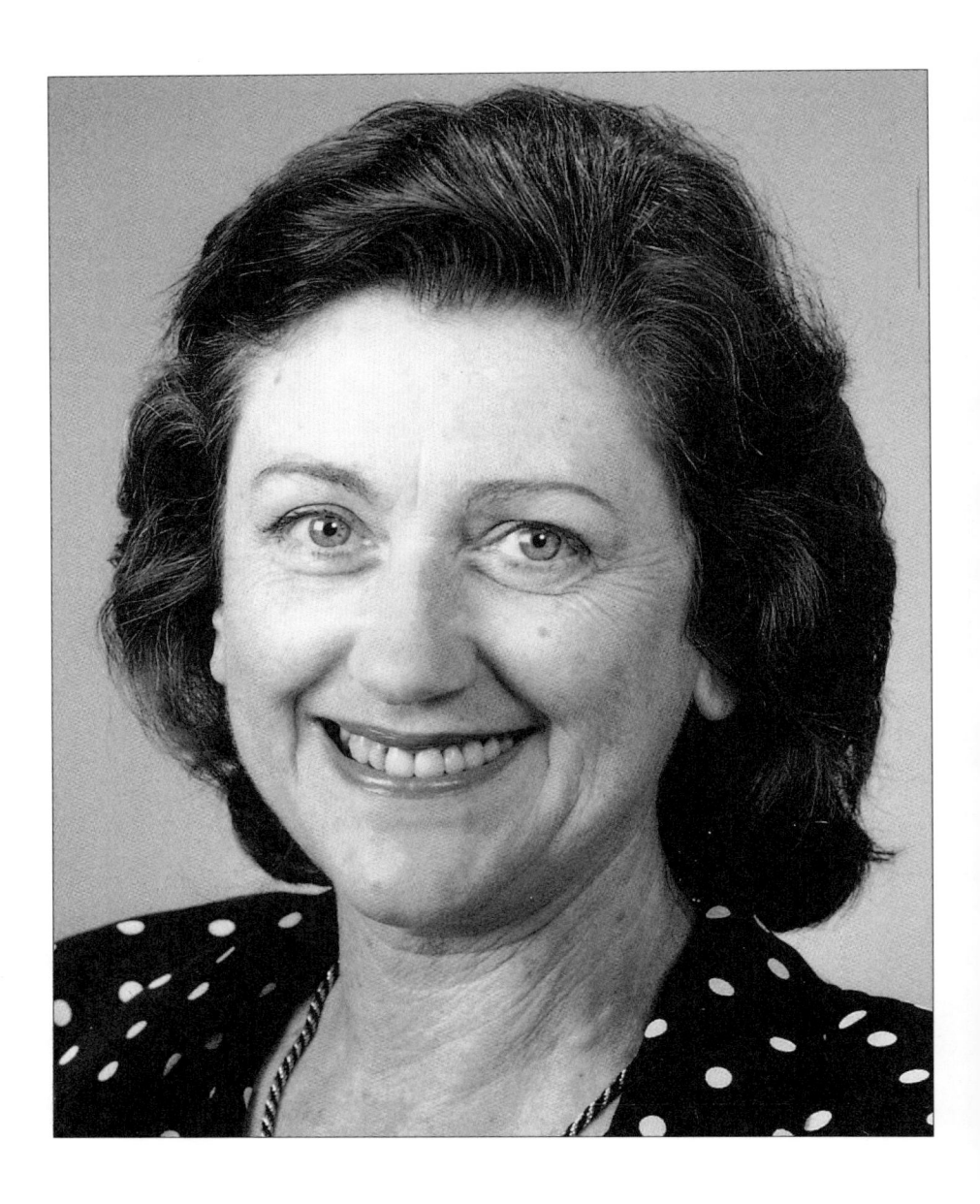

The reason I am pleased to be included in this book is because I became visible as an older woman in my fifties and I was invisible as a housewife.

❖ ❖ ❖

Jeannette McHugh

I drove to Jeannette McHugh's Marrickville office on a bright sunny day when gusty winds had dispersed any sign of the pollution one might have expected in her flat western Sydney electorate of Grayndler. Jeannette is a tall, slender woman with a lively intelligent face. Somehow the adjective 'soft' springs to mind. She has a soft voice, and softly curling brown hair; she moves gracefully and sits elegantly opposite me on the sofa, conceding that a preference for creating the conventional barrier by sitting behind her desk would intrude on our ability to build a rapport. But underlying the attractive femininity is a tensile strength, giving a glimpse of the toughness she must surely have to survive in the extraordinarily difficult, male-dominated world of federal politics.

Jeannette's story proved to be more apt to the theme of this book than I had anticipated. She is married to a justice of the High Court of Australia, Michael McHugh. Like Jeannette, Michael McHugh grew up in the industrial city of Newcastle in northern New South Wales. His early working life was spent in the rod-mill at the BHP, studying law at night through the Barristers' Admission Board course. He became one of the top barristers in Sydney before being appointed to the New South Wales Court of Appeal and, subsequently, the High Court. By any test his is an extraordinary success story and there can be no doubt that it is due to his prodigious talent and intellect. Nevertheless, it seems reasonable to assume that his road to the top was made easier because he had a partner who accepted responsibility for their home and three children. Until her late forties, Jeannette McHugh was the classic wife and mother. Like most women of her generation, she devoted herself to the family and did a bit of voluntary work on the side. In her case, the voluntary work happened to be in the local branch of the Labor Party – and, to her astonishment, in 1983, when she was forty-eight years of age, she was asked to run for parliament largely, she asserts, because everyone was so used to saying when they wanted something done, 'Oh, Jeannette'll do it.' Whilst such self-deprecation is clearly without foundation, nevertheless Jeannette's career, apart from her family, only happened on the threshold of her fifties.

Jeannette McHugh was the first woman from New South Wales to be elected to the federal parliament. She first represented the seat of Phillip, taking in Sydney's affluent and Liberal-voting Eastern suburbs as well as the more Labor-oriented south. It was the quintessential swinging seat which, before her succession, had belonged to the Liberals. Of course women have rarely been offered preselection for safe seats, a situation which is only now being recognised and steps taken to ensure fairer representation. Jeannette's election was a tribute to the hard work and personal characteristics she brought to the task. And she not only got elected, she also managed to hold the seat in later contests when the large swing to Labor during the early 1980s had dissipated, an obvious reflection of the regard which she built up among her constituents.

An electoral redistribution saw her seat abolished and she then successfully sought preselection for Grayndler, a Labor stronghold. In 1992 Jeannette became minister for Consumer Affairs, a position she still retains.

Apart from her passionate commitment to issues of social justice, Jeannette is dedicated to preserving the environment and is active in the anti-nuclear and disarmament movements. She also supports the arts and her early career as a teacher is reflected in her interest in education. She chaired the House of Representatives Standing Committee on Environment, Recreation and the Arts as well as being a member of several committees on communications, education, the environment, women and social justice.

Jeannette made the point during our meeting that the fact that she and her husband were both based in Canberra now was not as convenient as one might suppose. A little wryly, she said that early on she had thought that he could perhaps sometimes join her at Parliament House for a drink or a meal, an expectation which was rapidly dashed when he said that as a High Court judge he must maintain his distance from such a political environment. So, she says, he has had to learn to cook!

One of the striking things about Jeannette's electorate office is the pleasant, relaxed atmosphere emanating from a staff who are clearly devoted to their boss and dedicated to helping her serve her constituents as well as possible. Of course loyalty is not an unusual attribute in the staff of a politician but the other outstanding characteristic one notices in dealing with Jeannette's staff is their quite unusual level of courtesy and consideration. There is no hint of the arrogance that sometimes creeps into a minister's personal staff, the implication so often apparent that their boss is so busy and has so many competing demands on their time that agreeing to a request is the bestowing of a favour. There can be no doubt that this minister sees her role as one of service and that her staff reflect that accordingly.

The only time an (understandable) bit of collusion became evident was when her secretary interrupted about an hour into our meeting to say that another appointment was looming. Knowing how busy politicians genuinely are, I indicated that we could bring the interview to a close reasonably quickly, only to be informed with engaging candour that I shouldn't worry, this was a pre-arranged 'fake' interruption in case I proved to be awful!

✥ ✥ ✥

I grew up in a very industrial city, in Newcastle, and there were three of us, three girls, daughters of teachers. One of the significant features of my life was that after the age of seven, right through until the end of secondary school, I was always in an all-girls class and always taught by women, mostly single women, because that was the style. It meant that I had all these wonderful role models. It fitted the pattern more of a modern girl who would be in a private single-sex school. I was in the government system, and very proud of being in the government system, but even in the government system girls could be segregated.

It also had a bad effect on me in that being one of three girls, never mixing with boys at school, never being taught by a man, I thought that I would never understand men, that I would always be scared of them. I was certainly scared of boys and it is amazing that I have ended up in a job where most of my colleagues are men. I think it is probably only at this great age, in my fifties, that I have adjusted to that. Just by virtue of being surrounded by men now in my job all those original fears have disappeared but when I was a child they were real fears.

Those fears didn't disappear for a long time. Certainly I married and had children and two of them were boys, but I went teaching too and taught in an all-girls school in the government system. I taught for a couple of years in an all-girls school in the private system too, always surrounded by women. When I married I gave up work and was out of the paid workforce for twenty-three years being 'the housewife' at home with the children. I was the typical housewife so, for all those years, I didn't mix much with men. I'm not saying it was a preoccupation not mixing with men or the fact that I didn't understand them, but when I got a job I was surrounded by men, I was working with them, and it just came to me very easily. It was terrific. Of course, by then one has discovered a lot about them.

My father was an enormous influence on me, an absolutely enormous influence. We have discovered through our lives, the three girls, particularly in the last couple of years since his death, that he was an enormous influence on a lot of people. He was a schoolteacher and even now you can't go to Newcastle without every other person you meet having been taught by Charlie Goffet. So he was one of those people who had a great influence on me and it was quite profound.

It was he who encouraged us to achieve, perhaps without our realising that was what he was doing. Indeed, it was our mother who set more store by the fact that we had achieved something or other and I thought my father was always playing such things down. I remember embarrassing my mother terribly when she would make some modest boast in front of other people that I had won a prize or done something at school and I would rebuke her. What she did embarrassed me and I thought that she set great store by all this, whereas our father didn't. But it was quite obvious, looking back, that he was the one that expected us to do well. I remember coming home once after we had licked the enormous barrier of going from the little local suburban primary school to high school in town, and boasting to my father that I had done well. The only thing I had done badly in was maths — and he was thrilled to bits. That really showed the times. He was a languages teacher and he was extremely interested in English and languages. The mathematicians, the scientists, were the sort of people that went to the tech high rather than the high school where you learned Latin and French. What an influence that must have had on me. People are only now beginning to work out mechanisms to allow young women to excel at maths, for example, with things like separate classes because the girls can't show in front of the boys that they are good at what is alleged to be a boys' subject, although of course it is not. At any rate, I thought maths wasn't something for me to be in, I was going to please my father by doing well in all those good cultural things like languages, and I did.

My father was also a political influence. He was in the Teachers' Federation in the 1940s which was bitterly divided between the Left and the Right, which he referred to as the Communists and the Catholics. That is how it was defined in his terms.

As far as achievement goes, it was just taken for granted that the three of us would go through to the leaving certificate and on to university. It was also assumed that the only way you could afford that was to get a teachers college scholarship and teach. Young women in those days had few options other than teaching, and within teaching the majority taught English, history and languages. Everyone followed that pattern and a remarkable consequence of that is that my generation was taught by some of the most brilliant minds in Australia. Now, because the options are so varied, women are not necessarily choosing teaching and that's a shame because it should be acknowledged and esteemed as a great profession and it's not.

Because my parents were teachers we had advantages that all the kids around us did not have. I'm not sure whether to describe my childhood as a working-class childhood or not. We lived in a very working-class area right next to the BHP. The BHP was the major influence in my life. I just hated it. It was a powerful influence and a political influence. All the children I went to school with were the children of working-class parents who mainly worked at the BHP. Everyone we knocked around with was working class, we had our holidays every year at the little mining village of Redhead, my grandparents from the Cardiff area were as working class as you could possibly be. But we were the daughters of teachers and that made a big difference. If the BHP happened to be on strike I was the only one who would get the little lifesaving certificate because it cost sixpence. And there would be no doubt that I would be able to afford it. However, I am still more comfortable with working-class people and will be all my life.

I wasn't all that young when I married. It sounds young today, but in our day to wait until you were twenty-five to get married meant you were just about on the shelf. I was married when I was twenty-five and had my first child at twenty-six.

I had two children before our second wedding anniversary and I had left work. I had been teaching and I was earning probably twice as much as the man I married. It is an indication of those days too, that you wouldn't dream of not getting married if you were going to have children. You wouldn't dream of maintaining your single name. We did some pretty daring things at the time like rushing off and getting married without telling anyone except our parents, and doing it in a registry office. That was a bit radical but you wouldn't dream of just living together and I wouldn't have dreamed of saying, I am still Jeannette Goffet, even though I bitterly resented losing my name. I thought I was Goffet through and through. It is amusing that later, when I had become politically active, my husband, who by then was very high in his profession, said to me one night, 'I wish you would go back to using your maiden name, you are becoming an embarrassment,' and my reaction was to say, 'Certainly not.'

Those were the days when you had a career or a family. There was absolutely no question of doing the two. I had very romantic notions of what marriage would be like but it had never occurred to me that upon marriage I would lose completely the idea of a paid job. That came as a terrible shock to me. I had always thought that one day I would go on and be a university lecturer or ... I had extraordinary notions. I thought that one day I would learn to play the piano well and be a concert pianist, or that one day people would discover that I was a great actress. I had all these romantic notions and I don't think it ever occurred me, until it actually happened, that upon marriage and children, I gave up all that.

I did resent it but at the same time I thought it was just some terrible misfortune that had befallen me. Also, it coincided with the overwhelming job of being a mother. I never had time to think about the fact that I resented it because I was finding it totally consuming being a mother. Absolutely totally. I used to say at the end of the day, at the end of each day, well, I haven't managed to get any washing done but at least I have got dinner ready. I considered myself a total failure as a mother and a wife and I blame the *Women's Weekly*, the women's magazines, absolutely for that. Together, perhaps, with my own lack of preparedness. I had never cooked until the week I was married. So it is obvious that I had expected to be a woman who would do all those other achieving things and yet I had this very romantic view of marriage. I must have been crazy.

People often ask why I am described as 'housewife' in *Who's Who* and there are a few reasons for that. First, when I was first invited to be included as a member of parliament, I didn't want to go in it at all. I couldn't believe that I was a role model for other women, even though I spend a great deal of my time encouraging women, both middle-aged women and young women, to contribute to the political process because the political process needs women. Young women have got to understand it's where they should be and older women are an enormous untapped resource. But I couldn't see my own person as being a role model and so there was a dilemma — should I go in or not? I didn't want to. The way I got in was through Barry Jones [MP] and it was because of my mother. I resented it very much that when *Who's Who* sent you a draft entry it said that you were the daughter of your father and you had two sons and one daughter, even though the daughter was born first. Also, you married a man who was the son of a father and not a mother and I was outraged by that, that people are to assume that you have a father and no mother when the mother is the linchpin of the family situation, certainly the one that I was in. Barry Jones said, 'I notice that your husband is in *Who's Who* and you are not.' I told him why not and he said, 'Well, if I put the entry in, saying that you are the daughter of Charles Goffet and Neta Welsh, how would that be?' It is ironic that my wonderful mother who actually would have been so proud for us to be in *Who's Who* got us in there after she died.

The reason my occupation is given as 'housewife' is because I became politically active while I was in the unpaid, full-time job of being a housewife. From 1961, when I left teaching, I was doing the hardest work I had ever done in my life and, like all housewives, you do all these jobs but you are not paid to do any job, and therefore if you have to fill in a form you can't give an occupation. Even on the electoral roll you were then termed 'HD' — Home Duties. Don't think that didn't get me angry. One of the political jobs I was given was to be a member of Neville Wran's [former NSW Premier] first Women's Advisory Council. Every other woman on the Council was either a doctor or a teacher or a lawyer or a business person or had a job which was paid. My job was housewife. So I thought well, I'll say I'm a housewife — that's what I am. I realised after that when I became a member of parliament and they asked for my CV that what I had been doing for the last twenty-three years was being a housewife so I made quite a big thing of it. I get very cross when people say, you didn't work or, you didn't have a job. I can tell you that not once in all these years have I referred to a woman at home as not having a job or not being at work; it is just not paid.

I became politically active because in those days many more women were at home than in the paid workforce and they were the support for the government education system by way of the mothers club and the ladies auxiliary which were subsidiaries of the Parents and Citizens Association. I hope to heaven they have got rid of the words 'mothers club' and 'ladies auxiliary' now. They probably have, because they can't find enough mothers, not in the unpaid workforce, to do it. So I had to get involved and the first political activity for me was being taught how to sew a potholder for the fête. Not many years later I was one of those instrumental in getting rid of the fête because it was wrong that we had to raise money for public education to buy books and so on.

Once you get into an organisation, very soon, because you have the time, they make you secretary, and so you are writing letters to politicians because you need lights outside the school or whatever. You are involved in politics and I spend a lot of time pointing that out to women, that we are a wonderful resource for political decision-making because we understand so well how the system works. So really, I just got forced into it.

As far as joining the Labor Party was concerned, that came about because I had become very distressed, as most of Australia was, although they were not admitting it then, about the Vietnam War. I had actually started marching down the street. I realised even then that I had to make a political point even as I marched, which was to wear very shiny shoes and a neat suit so that when they called out from the footpath, 'Go back to Russia, you Commie poofter, long-haired...whatever,' I didn't fit the pattern.

I then determined in my isolation in the domestic scene — and isolation is the worst thing about it — that I had to belong to something. I had grown up a Labor voter and could not possibly not vote Labor no matter how bad the bastards were, so I joined the Labor Party and I am glad I did. The Labor Party, like all political parties, is built on the voluntary work of its branch members. My branch had the ideal volunteer in me, a woman at home with children, and they just kept giving me more and more jobs to do. Over the years political activity became an almost full-time, out-of-the-house activity.

I made the jump from voluntary activity to standing for election because someone pushed me. My story may not fit all women in their fifties, but it fits an awful lot of us. And it must not be the pattern for the future. I come from a very traditional era and I was continuing that in my own family situation. I slaved after them, I really did. I never thought I did it well enough. I had absolutely no self-esteem. Even though I had plenty of self-esteem as a child at school, all those years as a housewife knocked it out completely. I don't want to denigrate in any way at all the work of women at home, indeed, I want it to be acknowledged, praised and I want people to be grateful for it, I want society to thank women who do it. But I wasn't suited to it. Also, part of the attitude of women who were children in the 1940s was that you did any job as a volunteer. Plus, because of the way I had been brought up, to make the jump I was the sort of person who had to wait for someone to tell me to do it. I had been so busy all those years in the branch and had been sent off to do work on this committee and that committee and I think my colleagues were so used to saying, 'Oh, Jeannette'll do it,' that they said when they needed a candidate, 'Oh, Jeannette'll do it,' not realising that there had never been a woman from New South Wales in the federal parliament.

For more than eight decades since federation, New South Wales had never been represented in the federal parliament by a woman and that is extraordinary. The fact that the person who was actually there first was a middle-aged housewife of the Left probably needs some looking into.

It is the best thing that ever happened to me. It's been terrific. I would have to say that the fifties have been the best time of my life because it has been going back to being Jeannette again. There's no doubt about that. I remember being in a corridor in the old Parliament House one day, I was forty-eight or forty-nine, and it just suddenly dawned on me that I wasn't Mum. I couldn't get their dinner that night because I was in Canberra and they were in Sydney. It was like being back at school. Actually, Parliament House is really like a school, but it was a while before I realised that meant that I was Jeannette again. So the fifties for me are fabulous because to my astonishment and against all expectations Labor kept winning government and I kept winning the seat. So, whereas it was expected that I would be there in this very marginal seat for one term or two terms, I kept on.

It was extremely difficult for the family. I was lucky in that my electorate was the smallest in Australia and the nearest to Canberra so they didn't have to suffer as families of politicians often do but they had had me at home looking after them, no matter how badly, for a long time and it was an enormous shock to them. It was also an enormous shock to me. I felt guilty for a long, long time but that was balanced by my delight at being away from the responsibility of looking after them all the time. I always said they were very supportive but after a while I looked at it a little more honestly. I remember my youngest son saying when I once complained that they weren't much help, 'But Mum, we *let* you do it.'

The children are now, in their own way, very politically active. One son is a branch member in my electorate and my daughter once gave up an enormous amount of time to run one of the campaign offices, so they have in very specific ways been supportive in later years but I have got to say it was a shock to us all.

My husband used to say, 'I think that's terrific, Jeannette, you really should do it,' but the adjustments were pretty severe, they really were. I am not sure how well he has been able to come to terms with it. He is a man who is enormously supportive of the advancement of women in his particular field, enormously supportive, but he is of a generation which still expects the dinner to be on the table every night and I would say that it has been almost impossible for him to adjust to the fact that it is not going to happen. His mother serviced his family magnificently and totally and I tried for a long time. It is going to be different from now on for younger women. Younger women will expect a more sharing arrangement of the partnership.

I fitted in all the political activity to the domestic arrangements for many years. I think the shock was when it was going to take me out of the home and my family's reaction was, on the one hand, delight and 'good on you' and it was something that they might be able to boast about, but that was balanced by the obvious irritation that you just weren't there any more.

I didn't find the fact that parliament is a male environment a difficulty and I can only explain that by saying that I was just so excited by the whole process. It was the political activity that was the important thing to me. It was because of the political activity that I was there, not because of fighting the fellows.

When I look back on the last eleven years, I have certainly experienced extreme discrimination but I didn't realise it was happening. I have changed now but when people used to ask if there is any discrimination in political life I would say no, because we were all getting the same salary and the same amount of stationery and so on and therefore, as I saw it, we were all equal. But of course there was terrible discrimination going on all the time and it is still continuing. I don't know whether it was so subtle that I wasn't awake to it or it is just that because I am as old as I am and had copped so much for so many years, as women of my generation were expected to, that I just took it for granted.

Unfortunately, politics is still what people think it is, a power game, and I have always had perhaps the very naive view that it shouldn't be, that politics is actually to get a job done. It sounds so unbelievably trite but I think that if women were running the country, politics would probably be very boring because we would just get on with doing the job. Of course, there would still be personalities and some would want to lead and some not, but it is a game the boys play and to a certain extent, as a woman, you bugger that up.

I have learned a lot over the years. As a typical example, when you go to a committee meeting, everyone else in the committee is a man, and you make some statement and there is a terrible silence and you think, or at least a woman of my generation thinks, you stupid thing, Jeannette, why did you say it? For a long time, I always thought it was me. I didn't think it was because I was a woman. But then you go along to the same committee meeting the next week and one of the fellows puts up the same proposal and everyone agrees to it.

Another thing about being a woman of my generation is that you think, oh good, at least they're doing it. But you also learn from that. We do manipulate the fellows. If we want certain things done it is quite obvious that we have to allow them to think it was their idea. It happens all the time. That's why politics needs a lot of more women in there because they don't have to play all these silly games.

I really learned about discrimination when I found myself in the position of standing for a vacancy in the Ministry. I had never expected to be a minister because I think a back-bencher's job is so enormously rewarding and it is also terribly important. Governments are elected because people are doing good jobs on the back-bench. However, for all sorts of reasons I was putting my hand up to be minister. The effect on the fellows was extraordinary because they hadn't planned for me to put my hand up. Of course this is politics and in Labor that involves factions. One faction certainly didn't want me and even within my own faction I discovered that they had thought of someone else. Each day I think they expected me to say, 'Look, I didn't really mean it and of course someone else can have the job and that would be terrific.' But I just didn't say it and each day I was still there. It lasted about a week, the whole thing, and it was great because by then it looked as if they were discriminating against me because I was a woman. The women of Australia were getting pretty cranky and they were sending letters and so on. I kept on saying, 'Look, here it is, it's the fourth day and they still don't know what to do with me, it's the fifth day and they still don't know what to do with me.' I learned a lot from that. Men find it very difficult to cope with things not going the way they planned. We, as women, have learned to cope with everything going against plan. Absolutely everything, and we cope. So I stayed and it was good. But I learned a lot about men and it was discrimination against a woman. It happens all the time, and it is still happening now. Last night I noticed on television something which could well have been a joint press release by a male colleague and me, being *his* press release.

What you do about it depends on the reason you are doing it. I am not going to have a fight with a fellow just for my own kudos because it doesn't get anyone anything, but if consumers, whom I am representing at the moment, are going to benefit from my kicking up a fuss then I'll bloody well do it.

If we are to get more women in politics, first of all Australians have got to be less cynical about politics, they have got to understand that they can be involved and can make a difference. The reason women have been so good, the reason we do the job so well — and we really do — is because we are better accepted by the public. We don't fit the stereotype of the political system and a boys' game which has everything to do with power and nothing to do with just getting on with the job of running the country. Women have enormous skills in managing families and so on. They are good at the job. I generalise, but I do think women have a sense of responsibility. Politics means looking after other people, and the fact that women think, yes, it's actually my responsibility to look after them, is an extremely good attitude for politics. Of course, this is a woman in her fifties talking. Young women who have not been through the decades that my generation has been through, where women were expected to take sole responsibility, apart from financial responsibility, for the wellbeing of the family, may not have that view.

Young women have to be encouraged and helped and supported in getting into the parliament but it is terribly important that we do not forget that older women are an enormous resource. We have got to be very careful that older women, who have so much to offer, are still valued.

I also think it is extremely important for older women to be politically active on their own behalf. The Older Women's Network is terrific, they are just wonderful. But the reason I am pleased to be included in this book is because I became visible as an older woman in my fifties and I was invisible as a housewife. I was invisible at the shop counter, unless I made a nuisance of myself. I was invisible getting the children on to the bus. It is still a delight to me to realise that people have to take account of me because of the job I am in. I often say to women that I got my first paid job after twenty-three years, when I was about to be fifty. I am a good example. People can look at me and say, well, if she can do it, surely I can.

We have got to encourage older women with their experience to be active and I think they are, I really think they are. A lot of older women say that they now have the time and the freedom to be active and to make their own choices about what they do when they did not have those choices and they did not have that freedom while their children were at home. It's just terrific, actually.

I am a bit concerned that, because I have had this enormous opportunity which came to me as an older woman, I have got a very rosy view of the fifties. Apart from having a good time at school, which I loved, and gazing adoringly at my children in the odd moments when I could because I was usually too busy, the fifties has been the best time I ever imagined anyone could have in your life. I have this great job and when I am no longer a member of parliament, political activity will still keep me going. I will still be able to be politically involved as a much older woman.

I am ambivalent about getting older. I can see that it matters. For a start, people are surprised to find you are as old as you are. It is not because of the way you look. It is just because you are politically active or because you are doing all these things and enjoying it, they expect that you are a younger woman. It is all people's expectations and that is what we have to change.

On the other hand, how do you look at it? If you say, I'll be sixty next birthday, does that mean getting used to the idea that in ten years I will be seventy? Each one sounds a bit too old to cope with.

I have always been one of those people who has enormous highs and lows. I think we are all pretty emotional really and if we don't show it we are crazy. I don't find any lessening in that at all, quite the contrary.

I find older women are an enormous inspiration if they are fit and active. I have never been a person that kept myself beautiful but I have been very lucky in health and the idea of being a sick old lady or an unfit old lady fills me with absolute terror. However, the Older Women's Network is proving to older women that it is not automatically to be assumed that they will be sick or frail or any of those things. I have been lucky as far as health goes but I do now want to keep myself fitter.

Every time I see an old woman, and there are lots of them who travel and who are involved in everything and who are lucky enough to be healthy, I find that enormously inspiring.

PHOTO CREDITS

JAN BOWEN: *Jonathan Chester*
SARA HENDERSON: *David Hancock, Skyscans*
WENDY MCCARTHY: *Mike Lyon Photography*
KENDRA SUNDQUIST: *Mane Photo*
EVE MAHLAB: *Karl Schwerdtfeger*
HELEN LEONARD: *Elaine Odgers Norling*
QUENTIN BRYCE: Ita *magazine*
JEANNETTE MCHUGH: *Peter West, Government Photograhic Service*